HUMAN

HUMAN

VOICES OF

TOMORROW'S DOCTORS

Edited by Tolu Kehinde

Dartmouth College Press | Hanover, New Hampshire

Dartmouth College Press
© 2019 Trustees of Dartmouth College
All rights reserved
Manufactured in the United States of America
Designed by Mindy Basinger Hill
Typeset in Adobe Caslon Pro by Westchester Publishing
Services

For permission to reproduce any of the material in this
book, contact Permissions, Dartmouth College Press,
6025 Baker-Berry Library, Hanover, NH 03755; or email
university.press.new.england-author@dartmouth.edu

Library of Congress Cataloging-in-Publication Data

Names: Kehinde, Tolu, editor.
Title: Human: voices of tomorrow's doctors /
    edited by Tolu Kehinde.
Description: Hanover, New Hampshire: Dartmouth
    College Press, [2019] | Includes bibliographical
    references.
Identifiers: LCCN 2018050565| ISBN 9781512603330 (pbk.) |
    ISBN 9781512603637 (ebook)
Subjects: LCSH: Medicine — Anecdotes. | Physicians —
    Anecdotes.
Classification: LCC R705 .H79 2019 | DDC 610 — dc23
LC record available at https://lccn.loc.gov/2018050565

5   4   3   2   1

TO THE ONE

WHO INSPIRES DREAMS,

AND TO THE PEOPLE THROUGH

WHOM THEY HAPPEN

CONTENTS

FOREWORD

Five years ago, I was invited by NYU Medical School to be a Professor of Medicine in Medical Humanities. They wanted me to teach my novel *The House of God* as part of their offerings in the Humanities Master Scholars Program for students. I had never taught it, and doing so was a remarkable experience. I had been away from medicine for years, and suddenly found myself in the thick of it. Hearing the medical students discuss the novel, I was gratified and excited. At first, I hadn't grasped how *young* they seemed—the age of our daughter, just out of college. Their path toward being doctors was near the beginning, and I was touched by their smarts, fears, obsessive work, and sense of community.

Now we have *Human*—a grand, real, and inspiring collection of individual medical students and residents writing about their experiences in various forms, from poetry to essay—and it's brilliant. I've never read anything like it, in its breadth of concerns, its validation of effort and discipline, its internationalism (from many parts of the world), diversity, and also variety. The only way it could have come out so well was for the sensibility and hard work of the editor, Tolu Kehinde. Hats off to her, and to her affecting and fine poems, some of which are featured here.

In one of the reflections in the anthology, "Where Do Broken Hearts Go?" the writer focuses on her class being told by a professor that in medicine, one had to "leave your emotional baggage behind." While nothing could be further from the truth, the orthodox American medical system is still—*still*—often not understanding or valuing the humane that comes from our emotional truth, shared between doctor and patient, student and student, and in any good relationship. Even though the essays in this volume often focus on the medical trainee's fear and the difficulty of "learning to remember everything," that's actually the easier part of the path. With all the screens students and doctors now carry, they always have the information, even, one might say, the knowledge. The harder part is learning how to "be with" the patient, and "be with" each other, no matter what. That's difficult.

In fact, the screens at your fingertips mean that you don't have to remember information or knowledge, you can always click on it. But while you can always forget information or knowledge, *you never forget what you understand.* Studies show that we understand best what we learn in situations of "emotion." I still recall my very first patient—because I was so nervous, I attuned with all my emotional might. Think of where you were when you heard of 9/11, or the results of the 2016 election. You never forget those moments. Similarly, when you are in positions of responsibility as a house staff member, you never forget your mistakes, because you have "emotional baggage" that they carry for you—which is good, because you never make those mistakes again.

One of the most touching things in this daring and important volume is how much fear of failing the students have—because we are often focused on information, rather than on how we make good connections with our patients, our colleagues, and our loved ones. Everyone has the info, not everyone has the heart. That's why this volume, written from the heart, is not only elegant and valuable—hearts opened up—but also a cry from the real true path: being human in medicine.

Let me offer a little avuncular comfort.

On the path, the stressful rocky path to becoming a doctor, the danger is isolation, and the safety is in the healing power of good connection. Beware getting isolated. Hold your relationships tightly to your chest. Depression and suicide are high in our profession. Suicide is the ultimate isolation. Looking back, isolation was the most destructive force in *The House of God*. Isolation can kill you, and in hard times, moving into good connection and asking for help will keep you alive.

Learning to use the word "connection," or "the We," in our work can be helpful. Two quick new LAWS—which are useful not only in medicine, but in your outside life:

1. *Connection comes first.* For instance, taking the history of a new patient, if you connect, you will hear everything; if you don't connect, you won't hear anything.

2. *It's not just what you say or do, it's what you do say or do next.* Everyone makes mistakes in relationship, in trying to be in a We. (My favorite part in this volume is "Mistakes.") The ones who succeed in good relationships, be it in medicine or elsewhere, are those who, when they find themselves in a disconnect, move into it and then right through it, to a better connection. Admit errors. Hang in there.

Reading all these poems and essays and stories, I was terribly moved; sometimes, to sadness. I know how much pressure many students put on themselves. It's one thing to have pressure from an aforementioned Professor—fairly common in the big medical institutions. It's another thing to buy into that system, and put that pressure on yourself. You are the generation who have worked and worked before medical school, doing everything: cured cancer, saved countries, invented God knows what app, created great art. Trust yourselves, and your colleagues. Your resilience is remarkable—but don't tie it up in the tight anxious ball of "self." Especially when you are suffering, move, always, *toward* being with others, toward the We—not back into I, yourself. When you want to curl up and fight through your suffering alone, move in the exact opposite direction: toward caring others.

Remember: everybody suffers. The issue isn't suffering, it's how we walk through it. If we try to walk alone, tough it out, we will suffer more and spread more suffering around. If we, on the other hand, walk through it with others, with *caring* others—and that's where we come in as doctors, *that's our job*, we're there with patients at the most crucial times from birth to death!—if we ask for help from caring others, and if we as caring doctors help others through, we will not suffer as much, and not spread more suffering around.

Which brings us to your final challenge.

3. *Learn your trade, in the world.* Your patient is never only the patient, but the world—family, community, global warming, where their water comes from, where the garbage goes, and living through the current horrific and fractious, even hateful, condition of, and danger to, our Republic. Modern medicine in the United States is, on the one hand, great in its new treatments and cures. But our medical system is in dire shape for us doctors, because of two factors that are more and more inhumane: money and screens (electronic medical records—EMRs)—which means money and money (the screens are billing machines). These two factors prevent us doctors from being able to take good care of our patients and ourselves. We didn't train this hard to be data-entry clerks, spending sixty percent of our days in front of screens. Your generation has to take back our profession, resist the

injustice of money and money-billing machines, so we can once again have the face-to-face time and energy to be in human relationship with our patients.

The inevitable solution will be *to squeeze the money out of the machines.* (The best working example is the not-for-profit Veterans Administration [VA], with its government-run computer system—free of billing. And interoperable with all other VA systems across the country.) By doing this, the United States will join the other "civilized" nations to provide a national health care system, with screens to help treatment, not to make epic profits. Make that epic, Epic profits. This is *your* fight now, the key fight to keep the human in medicine. To reclaim your lives as doctors. Join together. Resist.

The writing in this book—enticing readers to emotionally sound truths about the medical journey—is a great start and a constant reminder. It should be required reading for all of the medical profession.

SAMUEL SHEM | MD, DPhil, Professor of Medicine in Medical Humanities at NYU Medical School | July 14, 2018

INTRODUCTION

I often tell people that medical school has been one of the most challenging periods of my life, and emotionally more so than academically, although my test scores might tell you that it hasn't exactly been a walk in the park in that regard either. I came to medical school after a fantastic gap year in Boston, where I had met and built a strong community of friends that turned into a family of sorts. Consisting of mostly women—attending a women's college leaves you with a strong affiliation and love for women—my Beantown crew were the people with whom I explored my new city, the people in whose houses I had spare toothbrushes and designated pajamas, people with whom I discussed theology and explored tough questions about God and Christianity during our onesie-wearing "estrogen parties." These were the people who supported and prayed for me as I embarked on the almost year-long process that is medical school applications, and that came en masse to celebrate with me at my white-coat ceremony, complete with silly selfies and obligatory jumping pictures. And yet, these were exactly the ones I found myself without as I tackled eight-hour lecture days, biweekly tests covering textbooks worth of material, and declining sleep.

Prior to medical school, I had attacked every new opportunity with intense optimism and confidence, the kind that looked arrogantly ahead without even a last glance at the past. It wasn't that I did not cherish memories or the people that featured fondly in them, it was that I had developed a track record of immediate thriving even after the most heartfelt of goodbyes. I expected medical school to be challenging, especially academically, because everyone tells you it is. But I also expected to meet its challenge with a good work ethic and consequently, excel immediately at it. And so medical school said, "I'll raise you one, *chica.*"

I don't remember if there was ever one breaking point, one moment where I decided that it was too much, that I was done. Instead, I remember several breaking points, several towel throw-ins, several moments where tears were shed at the most mundane of stimuli. I also remember that it was in these moments that emotionally laden words collided into sentences in my brain and rolled off my thumbs unto my phone's notes app: I found poetry. One of my first poems came to me as I listened to a physician talk about his work with the homeless population in Boston at a public health event. I was inspired by his life's work and encouraged by the fact that there was indeed meaning after the drudgery of medical school. But I was stuck on the in-between: how does one nurture dreams of a far-off promised land, and yet live contently in the realities of a current one that devitalizes? So I wrote:

> Your belly burns
> with dreams so fierce,
> they convince you
> tomorrow will be lit
> almost entirely by their flames.
> But tomorrow is still tomorrow.
> Today, you must face the reality
> that on a cold day,
> imagined fires are scarcely enough.

The poems never really provided answers to my questions or completely resolved my angst about the path I was on, but they served as outlets for my emotions in an environment that often treats emotion as taboo. They soothed me with the comfort that comes from creating, from knowing that you can bend shapes and words, in a way that sometimes brings beauty amidst uncertainty. Poetry thus became my fortress, and also the means through which I rebuilt my social system: it became a way to tell the world—read: small group of Instagram followers—that I was struggling quite a bit, that medical school isn't all that it is cracked up to be or, perhaps put differently, that it is all it is cracked up to be and then some. Putting myself out there in words made it easier to reach out to people around me: classmates, other medical students, family, my Beantown crew. I found that I was not alone, that my classmates were going through similar struggles and semi life crises, and that drawing on the strengths of people and experiences from times past was essential for survival. Indeed, a woman—particularly one in medical school—is not an island.

My story of survival—or surviving, because *sista* hasn't graduated yet—will not be complete without mentioning Lola, my cousin-sister-friend, who, despite working on a PhD, managed to provide a listening ear on days when tears fell freely, and serve as first reader for everything I wrote. We have always been close, but the past years have drawn us even closer in a way that has been life saving for me. Through her constant cheerleading and friendship, I have found small ways to nurture dreams of a far-off, promised land, and yet live contently in the realities of a current one that *threatens* to devitalize. This book in your hands is one of these ways.

Like the poems I've written over the past couple of years, *Human* came out of a place of both introspection and reaching out: looking inward and writing about my own experience encouraged me to connect with other people around me. Medical training is a process of tremendous vulnerability. The human body is a complex machine for which mastery of the individual parts is as important as mastery of the whole. At the beginning of their training, learners are only vaguely aware of the impossibility of the task they have taken on but in part, because of the personalities drawn to careers in medicine as well as their previous triumphs in other academic settings, they approach the task with the mindset of complete conquest: all can be, and will be, known. And thus, from this point on, vulnerability becomes a steady companion. Very early, learners become acquainted with their limitations: all cannot, and will not, be known. An astute learner will also quickly realize that she is surrounded by incredibly brilliant minds and as she does, her own brilliant mind, which her uncle has bragged about to his friends for as long as she can remember, will start to seem dull. And so she will push herself even harder — because *grit* — dispensing of seemingly inefficient uses of time: sleep, food, friends, sometimes family.

A study of students at a US medical university in 2013 found that the prevalence of major depressive disorder and generalized anxiety disorder among medical trainees are about five and eight times higher than in age-matched controls. Similar trends also occur in other countries around the world: studies in Canadian and Pakistani students in 2016 showed significant psychological distress in a subgroup of medical students. Another 2015 paper reviewing studies from 1990 to 2015 also found a high prevalence of burnout among medical trainees internationally, with some studies finding high emotional exhaustion in thirty-five to forty-five percent of medical students. Unfortunately, this pattern continues into residency, with levels of depersonalization — feeling detached from patients — and burnout increasing. Worse, the American Foundations for Suicide Prevention also estimates that 300 to 400 physicians die by suicide per year in the US (at the time of writing, just this month, a medical student and psychiatry resident, both affiliated with a New York medical community, died by suicide within a week of each other). These trends are particularly concerning considering matriculating medical students appear to start out with higher quality of life scores and lower burnout and depression rates than controls. Something happening during medical training seems to be tipping the scale.

Whatever it is, a lot of students go through it alone. Suffering in silos, students rarely talk about their struggles. In my first two years at medical school, the few times I heard anything close to vulnerability from my classmates were during our weekly "On Doctoring" groups. These groups, consisting of seven to eight students and a physician facilitator, were designed to teach the basics of doctoring to first- and second-year students. However, our facilitator—God bless her—always started our sessions with what I call "feeling sessions." We would go around the room and talk about what was going on in our lives—read: complain about school—and once in a while, she would ask one of us, "So how does that feel in your body?"

I started *Human* as an attempt to answer that question honestly and get other medical trainees to do so too, because looking inward, for me, has been a fundamental part of forging ahead. As I solicited reflections over the course of my third and fourth years, I hoped the anthology would go beyond the commonly scripted anecdotes and capture what it really *feels* like to be in medical training: mentally, physically, emotionally, and spiritually. I wanted the anthology to focus on the trainees—medical students and residents—themselves, not patients or anyone else (although, as you will see, this is hard to do since the people we care for sometimes define who we are), because in learning to recognize and preserve the dignity and humanity of others, medical trainees often forget their own. I wanted *Human* to be a reminder to medical trainees that we matter, we are not alone, and that, even on this road to Doctor, where it seems like our lives are on hold, we are living and evolving.

I also hoped *Human* would not just highlight the individual's efforts on the path to Doctor, but would also emphasize the path as a communal one. Very few people make it through medical training solely by their own efforts (I don't think anyone does really, but I'll leave room for the rare exceptions). Yes, it is the individual that sits through hours of often mind-numbing lectures and spends even more hours memorizing every detail of these lectures. It is also this same individual that writes the numerous examinations that litter the path to Doctor, often burdened by increasing debt and, sometimes, declining health. However, all this is made possible by that friend that sends those YouTube videos of narcoleptic goats (sometimes during those mind-numbing lectures, and thank God for this) and by the parent that sends a daughter home with a month-supply of cooked food so she doesn't have to subsist on Ramen while she studies. The path is paved by that generous mentor that offers to pay for a required standardized exam (because, let's face it, medical student is often synonymous for no money) and the cousin that offers to call in fifteen minutes, because power naps can be magical except for when they extend till the next morning and test materials have not been reviewed. For community members, I hope *Human* shows the part you can play in medical education: your support is vital for producing healthy, whole physicians. I hope it also shows you just how human, like you, your doctors are.

The reflections you are about to read consist of essays, poems, and quotes from medical students and residents across the world. When I started working on *Human*, I was armed simply with an idea, pent-up emotion and a laptop. Unsure about how to get the word out, I was naïve enough to think that emailing every medical school dean and university administrator across the world would do the trick. Somehow, it worked! Although I never got responses to many of my emails, I received several congratulating me on starting the project and offering to pass word about *Human* on to their trainees. After hearing about the project through one of my emails, one trainee sent me a compilation of her classmates' quotes she had been amassed over her first year at medical school. The quotes embodied the raw emotion I wanted captured in the anthology—so much so that most chapters in *Human* begins with one of these quotes.

In soliciting reflections, I asked my colleagues to think deeply and honestly about their own experiences in medicine. I asked them to consider the ways in which they have changed through, and because of, medical training. In editing the responses I received, I have tried to maintain my colleagues' voices, emotions, and intents as much as possible, even up to retaining the British spellings of contributors living outside the United States. Similarly, in reference to real people and events, some contributors have chosen to maintain real names. Others have chosen to conceal them. I upheld all such choices in editing the anthology. I have also chosen to maintain a diversity of form— poetry, prose, quotes, lists—in this anthology to underscore the unique ways in which trainees experience medicine. While the anthology doesn't cover all that the trainee experience entails, it does shed more light on the internal workings of medical trainees and cover a sufficient array of topics to facilitate productive discussion. *Human* will not be a silver bullet in the conversation about how our societies train their doctors, but I hope it will contribute meaningfully to the dialogue.

You will notice that I have chosen not to include full names after each reflection (although contributors' full names do appear immediately following this introduction). I chose this format because while these reflections are personal, many of the sentiments within them are shared by many trainees across the world. I want the experience of reading *Human* to be one in which readers go through the book seamlessly, seeing themselves and their experiences within the reflections, without anchoring too much on who wrote what. I hope by doing this I have not taken any credit away from the anthology's contributors or their experiences.

As you read the reflections, I hope you are able to truly able to sit with some—or all—of them and find parts that you can identify with, whether you're in medicine or not.

REFERENCES

Brazeau CM, Shanafelt T, Durning SJ, et al. Distress among matriculating medical students relative to the general population. *Acad Med.* 2014;89(11):1520–1525.

Dyrbye L, Shanafelt T. A narrative review on burnout experienced by medical students and residents. *Med Educ.* 2016;50(1):132–149.

Imran N, Tariq KF, Pervez MI, Jawaid M, Haider II. Medical students' stress, psychological morbidity, and coping strategies: a cross-sectional study from Pakistan. *Acad Psychiatry.* 2016;40(1):92–96.

Matheson KM, Barrett T, Landine J, McLuckie A, Soh NL, Walter G. Experiences of psychological distress and sources of stress and support during medical training: a survey of medical students. *Acad Psychiatry.* 2016;40(1):63–68.

Mousa OY, Dhamoon MS, Lander S, Dhamoon AS. The MD Blues: Under-Recognized Depression and Anxiety in Medical Trainees. Courvoisier DS, ed. *PLoS ONE.* 2016;11(6):e0156554. doi:10.1371/journal.pone.0156554.

CONTRIBUTORS
(In Order of First Appearance)

Bryan Pham
Ianna Hondros-McCarthy
Tahireh "Rae" Shams
Luke Austen
Mofiyinfoluwa Obadina
Nara Michaelson
Katherine Ferguson
Tolu Kehinde
Sonal Kumar
Cameron Sadegh
Lye-Yeng Wong
Benjamin Doolittle
Vanessa Soetanto
Mbulelo Koko
Stephanie Wan
Andrew Huang
Jennifer Fleischer
Tina Jaramillo
Alexandra Houston-Ludham
Erik Andrews

Ashley Hamel
Habsita Abakar
Gideon Mutai
Kayla Simms
Uchechukwu Osondu
Natalie Ring
Jihan Ryu
Sherry-Ann Brown
Marina Malak
Sarah Hanafi
Daphne Doble
Caledonia Buckheit
Glara Rhee
Moira Haggarty
Olubunmi Akintola
tammi cooks
Diane Brackett
Joshua Jolissaint
Nayan Agarwal
Ene Morgan

Peace Eneh

Gloria Onwuneme

Katherine Brooks

John Mascari

Riddhi Desai

Sahil Batra

Takudzwa Ngara

Afolabi Boluwatife

Mariah Robertson

Samuel Brunwasser

Faith Robertson

Christina Georgeades

Maxime Billick

Amir Meiri

Sheree Brown

Trevor Morey

Megan LaPorte

Dr. Mikey

Anna Duncan

My-Linh Nguyen

Syed Shehab

Vikar Singh

Barbara Salas

June Garen

HUMAN

ONE

FIRSTS

> I have a bucket for soaking formaldehyde-soaked
> scrubs in my apartment.
>
> *Anonymous*

*Medical training offers an array of firsts, whether it's delivering
a baby for the first time or a first overnight shift. The reflections
in this chapter focus on the emotions that punctuate trainees' first
few days and months in medical school or residency. They also
highlight what happens when the novelty of once-special moments
begins to wear off.*

Unforgettable

Plastic coverings were removed,
towels placed, precise incisions made.
It didn't seem all that bad, just another lab.

Right?

Who did I just cut into?

BRYAN P. | United States

The Blank Slate of Delivery

"They'll be making the incision any minute. Want to come in with me and learn how to catch a baby?" I wondered if this huge blonde presence in navy scrubs had any idea how cool I thought that would be — to be in the same room when a whole new person took their first breath. I had a feeling she knew exactly how cool it was, and that had probably been the driving force of her choosing this profession.

"Since this is your first time, you can just watch today, and maybe you can catch the baby tomorrow," she said, as we walked down the calm hardwood hallways with floral and landscapes decking the beige walls. She dwarfed me, and I felt a little like an eager rabbit hopping along, giddy at my good fortune. She handed me a hairnet, booties to put over my shoes, a face mask, and a blue jacket to wear into the OR; I wouldn't be fully scrubbed in like she would be, and I liked that better — no one could accidentally expect me to do anything.

"You can stand against the wall over there — by the foot of the bed, where you can see everything happening," she said, as she went to make sure everything was set up for the baby once it was pulled out of the mom's uterus. I felt like I was in an exhibit, enthralled by the artistry and ingenuity I was witnessing. The surgeon was already at work, with about five assistants surrounding him. My eyes felt like tea saucers as I watched people pulling back the skin from the gaping circular hole in the mother's abdomen with giant spoons. You could see the grape-like clusters of yellow fat, and the cellophane-like fascia the surgeon was deftly separating away. They were going down into the abdomen layer by layer, cauterizing blood vessels to stop bleeding along the way, so that everything was clear. It was an organized procedure I was watching, not a messy gore. Still, I was glad for the wall at my back as I felt the familiar queasiness of surgery. It had been a while since I'd passed out, but the comfort wasn't there, and I was immensely glad not to have the responsibility of making a person's very first experience not be being dropped on an OR floor.

I smiled with my eyes at anyone who looked at me, as the rest of my face was covered in sky-blue plastic. Some nurses came and explained things, and I hoped they were happy to see the gratitude on my face. I hoped it reminded them a little of just how insanely cool it was to be present at a baby's first cry into a foreign medium. I wondered if something like that were to happen to an adult, if it would feel like falling through into a fourth dimension like Einstein's string theory.

The surgeon took what looked to me like two giant plastic embroidery circles with a tube of cellophane linking them, and inserted it into the mother's abdomen, further retracting all the layers he had just worked his way through, leaving the fleshy bowling ball of her uterus in clear view. It looked a little like a rose marble flecked with dark purples and light yellows, but mostly a dusty-rose color. The surgeon lightly scraped a horizontal line into the uterus with a scalpel while an assistant followed with suction to keep everything clear. He passed over that same line over and over again, nice and lightly, so as not to cut too deep to nick the baby a few centimeters below. All of a sudden, he was opening the incision with his fingers, and you could see the thin matted black hair over a tiny, oblong skull. Immediately after, the head popped out, followed by a body and an umbilical cord that made me think of those long, twisted lollipops. The little girl started a gurgly cry immediately, and I was grinning hard under my mask, because crying meant her lungs worked! It meant she was alive! It meant she had a great chance at becoming the amazing human being she already was!

The physician's assistant (PA) was there with a white, teal, and burgundy striped blanket, deftly holding the baby in her arms as she brought her over to a side table to continue rubbing her body to make her cry, and therefore breathe. The PA suctioned the fluid that had previously been both the baby's source of nutrition and excretion of urine out of her mouth, then her nostrils, encouraging a completely new way of life for her. I couldn't believe how clean she was! There was barely any blood on her writhing little blue body, and she just had the tiniest, perfect finger and toenails! Her belly button was still a fleshy canal that the lollipop of her umbilical cord plugged into. Her eyes just barely peeked open, and I felt bad for all the bright lights barraging her. I was glad that she hopefully had yet to even understand anger or forgiveness, so couldn't make anything of the discomfort other than it being that—a pure, unadulterated discomfort, devoid of a label of good or bad. The PA swaddled the baby and gave her to her father, and then left the room, with me regretfully following behind. I peppered her with questions and gratitude for the next twenty minutes, and she seemed to appreciate it. When she told me why she chose neonatal care as a profession, circles closed and the gears of my teeth clicked together in harmony.

"I fell in love with the blank slate of delivery."

IANNA H-M. | United States

Staying Alive

Just five short weeks into my first year of medical school, I was shadowing in the ER. I had never really considered myself a good fit for the ER, but I thought I'd never know for sure until I tried. Everything was new and exciting and I understood next to none of what was happening around me, save for the odd word here and there. Joined at the hip to my preceptor, I hopped from room to room clad in my white coat, trying to think like a doctor. I had shadowed this preceptor twice before, so I was eager to show that I had, in fact, learned something since our last encounter. To my dismay, I still met many of his questions with a "deer-in-the-headlights" stare. Fortunately, a resident was also with us, and shared the attention for most questions.

I hadn't been there too long before a code came in. An obtunded patient, Ms. Smith,* had been brought in by EMS. We rushed to the code room, where I picked a nice corner to stand in so I could be out of the way. The staff moved swiftly about the room like performers in a choreographed dance I'd missed all rehearsals for. I wanted to be useful, but I didn't even know what that would entail and asking didn't really seem feasible. I wasn't sure what to do with myself so I grabbed gloves and put them on—just in case (that's what doctors do, right?). I wore them for a while and realized I must look silly since I wasn't even near the patient, so I took them off. But then what if I was needed? And repeat. My preceptor hovered busily over Ms. Smith, calling out to me every so often to explain things. I nodded, despite understanding very few of the words he said.

The code lasted several hours, with Ms. Smith frequently crashing and requiring CPR. As if on cue, a line-up of nurses would form; they would take turns doing chest compressions until she was stable again. After a few repetitions of this cycle, I could see the nurses stretching and shaking out their arms in line. I had taken a CPR course a few weeks prior, so I technically knew what to do. I offered to help, explaining quickly that I'd never actually done it on a real person before. The nurses ushered me into the line and I glanced at my preceptor for approval. He looked, but continued what he was doing so I took that as a go-ahead. When I was next up, I'm sure I was visibly shaking. I kept thinking of how I'd never been able to get the practice dummy's "good CPR" indicator click to sound during my course, which did nothing for my confidence.

The moment in which I took my turn and stepped up on the stool next to Ms. Smith is burned into my mind. I felt all the blood drain from my face and, for a second, I thought I might pass out. I started chest compressions, singing "Stayin' Alive" in my head, to make sure I had the right beat. I was relieved that

* Name has been changed for privacy.

the patient was intubated because there is no way I could have counted the compressions. I kept going until my back ached and I could feel my compressions getting weaker, then I switched off. My preceptor told me I "did some good CPR," and I tried not to beam too much. After that, Ms. Smith stabilized for a while so we went to speak with her family. Her husband was in the code room with us, which is not how they do it on *Grey's Anatomy*, so naturally, I was surprised. I wanted to talk to him but I didn't know what to say, so I would just smile a little—but not too much—every time I caught his gaze.

Ms. Smith continued to crash for most of the day, until she passed away during a code. There were already enough doctors and staff in there so I wasn't in the room when it happened. The words were never explicitly said, at least not that I heard. I eventually had to ask. I was in disbelief, even though I shouldn't have been. I just felt like she would get better. I had no good reason to feel that way, but I did. I was shaken. It's difficult to describe the feeling. I had never had to deal with it before.

When the shift was over, I sat down to debrief with my preceptor. I was trying to be tough and stoic even though I could feel my eyes welling up. I tried to keep my answers short so as not to rattle the floodgates. We were talking about other things when he suddenly excused himself and came back with a box of tissues for me, which was unfortunately just enough to let the tears out. I was embarrassed about crying which, of course, just made me cry more. He was kind and gave me some advice on how he handled these things, and told me not to be embarrassed (though I still was). I thanked him, collected myself, and drove home.

Since beginning medical school, I have experienced some of the most memorable feelings I have ever had in my life. And it's only been six months.

RAE S. | Canada

The Sound of Silence

"Want to learn how to certify a death?"

"Yeah, please," I respond, remembering the tick box in my medical school log book next to "Certification of death and writing a death certificate." I immediately feel guilty for having done so. But all medical students know to take offers of teaching whenever they appear, even when it is related to the rituals around a patient's death.

James, one of the junior doctors on the general medical ward I am attached to, leads me down the ward and into a side room. The lights are off, the room dimly lit by the dull Thursday morning sky outside, and as I look down at the elderly woman dressed in her hospital gown, there is a stillness around us that I've never felt before. The radio on the bedside TV is still on . . . "It's 10:30 a.m. and we've got more great tunes coming your way, plus another chance to win . . ." This station's mood dial is permanently set to upbeat happiness which, in the current circumstance, now strikes me as bizarre.

"What do you think we have to do?" asks James.

"I know we need to listen to her chest . . ." I say.

"Yes, that's right, and there's more too."

James walks me through everything, step by step. First, he gently touches a rolled-up piece of tissue to the woman's cornea, the transparent outer layer of the eye.

"That would make me or you blink," James says, before shining a pen-torch in each of her eyes. Her pupils are still.

For the last reflex, he applies pressure to the bony grooves above the eyes. Nothing.

"Now you can listen to her chest."

I unwrap the stethoscope from my neck, and as I approach, I properly contemplate the woman in front of me for the first time. I am twenty-two and have seen death in many forms: the trauma of a middle-aged father unable to be resuscitated after more than an hour of chest compressions, the gory autopsy of an overweight man in the basement mortuary, and the plasticised, formaldehyde-covered body parts on the tables of the dissection room. But this is different. She is dressed like all the other patients, positioned in bed like all the other patients, but at some point this morning, her body overcome with disease, she stopped.

I pause, place my stethoscope on her chest, and listen.

"Who will be in this week's Big Top 40? Tune in to find . . ."

James steps round to the other side of the bed and turns it off. I listen again, and hear noises. Confused, I realise that my hand is trembling and that this is generating the interference I am hearing in my stethoscope. I steady myself, and there is nothing. Stethoscope anchored on her chest, where my ears are used to the rushing in and out of whooshing air and the rhythmic lub-dub, lub-dub of the heart, I hear the sound of silence. It is deep and unsettling.

To confirm death, doctors must listen to the chest for four minutes. As I listen, I briefly wonder who this woman was, where she called home, where she used to run around and play as a child. The time passes slowly, but it ticks by and I am done, and now James listens. We finish, and carefully pull the sheet up to her neck, as though tucking her into bed, and exit the room.

We emerge into the hustle and bustle of the main ward.

"What did she die of?" I ask.

"Heart failure and pneumonia," he replies. James documents the confirmation of death in the patient's notes, and then almost immediately is off, cracking on with the usual mountainous job lists created on the morning ward round.

At the end of a long life, death needn't be a defeat for doctors, more a natural result of medicine's limitations and the inevitable march of disease. But as I take out my logbook, I reflect on how much more difficult confirming death might be if the patient were younger, or the circumstances more tragic. I hadn't met the patient in life, which made things easier, but doctors are required to confirm death for patients they've cared for over weeks, months, or years.

I tuck the log book back into my pocket. Learning to acknowledge death is going to take more than a tick-box.

LUKE A. | United Kingdom

This piece was originally published in The Guardian Healthcare Professionals Network.

Transitions

I woke up too damn early, but I've done this before.
I drove down with my headlights on, music blasting, coffee
   steaming. I've done this before, many times in fact.
I got my list and figured out how to squeeze by everyone, in
   time. This isn't new to me.
I wrote my notes and presented my shaky plans. As I've done
   in the past.
I made my rounds, gave updates and followed up. Again,
   nothing new.
I added admits to my list. I hadn't done as often, but there's
   some experience.
But discharge . . .
Ending this complicated relationship, breaking this made-up
   simulation;
Ending this intrusion, and returning power to its rightful
   owner:
That was new.

MOFIYIN O. | United States

My First Patient

When you step into the anatomy lab for the first time, the thing that strikes you most strongly is the smell. But this quickly dissipates. A much more powerful sense takes over. Not one of sight or sound but more a combination of all your senses at once. As you look around at the black plastic bags resting quietly upon clean steel tables, you become immediately aware of your own existence. It is a difficult feeling to describe. You will unzip the bag apprehensively and there, completely nude, exposed to you in the most profound way, is another human. Someone who gave themselves for your education, someone who wished their body could be a tool that you would use to build your foundation of knowledge as a doctor. At that moment, there is nothing you are more grateful for and no one you have more respect for than that person lying in front of you. But that changes.

As the dissection continues, the body gradually loses its form and is reduced to something almost unrecognizable. The human lungs, the heart, the muscles, the nerves, now only serve academic functions. You begin to grow further distant from that feeling you felt when you first started. The body's fascias become hindrances to your understanding of muscle attachments, the nerves and all their branches become complex jumbles you wish were simpler, the blood clotted in the veins is removed as nonchalantly as you would remove walnuts from your salad, and the lab itself becomes an obstruction to your Friday night plans with your friends. It becomes a nuisance, just another thing you must get through to pass this stage.

I've always seen myself as a good person, or at least as someone who has always tried to find a way to do the right thing for the right reasons. A need for true satisfaction in life had pulled me down the medical path. I wanted a career with meaning and purpose, one that regardless of the hard work would leave me feeling content within myself. Knowing that my hands had worked tirelessly to relieve the burden of disease from a fellow human being seemed to me to be the only true path to fulfill that want. I could never work a job just for money and I never thought I could ever become numb to the sensation of someone else's need. But my yearlong study of human anatomy didn't fit the expectations that I had set for myself. I always thought of those physicians who cut out early or who were short with patients as terrible people who picked the wrong profession. I could never become like them because I knew myself—I was a good person with good intentions. But through the course of anatomy lab, I had come to understand just how a person could become one of "those people."

At the end of the year, I got to hold my cadaver's brain. It struck me that an entire human's life, memories, hopes, thoughts, and dreams were nestled in the palm of my hand. Perhaps one of those hopes would have been that I would respect and honor my lab experience and the sacrifice made for my learning. That moment was humbling: I had accomplished the academic task put before me, but still felt like, in some way, I had failed. But as I have pondered the whole experience more, I've realized that maybe I had in fact learned the greatest lesson that this person could ever have taught me: the need to be more self-aware and be grateful for the experiences I've been afforded so far in my education and life. If I can hold on to that feeling, I think I will have learned what it means to be a good person, just trying to do the right things for the right reasons.

ANONYMOUS | United States

First Night Shift

2:51 A.M.
First night of nights . . . did I listen to my body? I mean, possibly, but honestly, no . . . because if I did listen, I would be tucked under my blankets in my bed. I did eat, I mean, if you really

want to call that late night cafeteria food food . . . kinda delusional but not really . . . I'll decide when I really feel giddy. But in all fairness, this all seems like a cosmic joke, here I am diminishing my own health . . . food/sleep/beauty/youth. But I like to think it is not in vain. I did just get to witness birth. This time, I noticed I didn't cry from the overwhelming beauty of the process . . . I felt happiness but it kinda frightened me. Did I become what I judged in others or is it a normal human reaction to become desensitized to the overwhelming emotional rollercoaster of witnessing life come into the world? I remember noting how unphased my residents seemed during other births. I had tried to hide my emotion then, thinking it made me look weak.

I don't want to be cynical.

ANONYMOUS | United States

Code Blue

"Code Blue, room 1215," rang out over the speakers at 6:30 a.m., while we were organizing ourselves to trade off to the morning team of hospitalists, residents, and medical students. Ken and I ran down the two flights of stairs to room 1215. Every other time I'd done this, it had been a false alarm; this time there was dark greenish-black bile tracing from an elderly woman's mouth, framing the left side of her pale head on the pillow. She wasn't moving or breathing. Her face was ashen with closed eyes.

"Start compressions," our attending said, and a big male nurse started, one knee up on the bed to get better leverage to bear straight down on her heart, putting in the muscle to get it to pump from the outside now. As he jack-hammered away at a rate of 100 compressions per minute, I watched as more bile pumped out of her mouth. Her stomach had herniated up through her diaphragm and was sitting around her heart, rather than below it. So he was pumping blood out of her heart and bile out of her stomach at the same time. Another nurse was bringing a bag-valve mask to the head of her bed to deliver oxygen into her lungs, but I could see her hesitating. The bile was coming up out of the patient's mouth and she had breathed some of it into her lungs—that's what had caused her heart to stop. Her lungs had gotten filled up with fluid, so oxygen couldn't get into her blood, and the heart muscles that depend on oxygen could no longer work. The nurse knew this, and maybe she was wondering, like I was, if pushing air into the lungs might also push more fluid in there. But it didn't matter—in order for her to have any chance of getting her organs working again, she needed air, so air she got, with a small allowance on the side for bile to leak out past her cheek.

The jackhammering arms had slowed, now two minutes into CPR, and I could tell they weren't right on top of the middle of her sternum anymore. "Stop compressions and take a carotid pulse," our attending said. The nurse put his finger to the woman's neck as a technician applied defibrillator pads to the woman's chest. The nurse shook his head and took a pair of scissors of out his pocket, cutting away her black-smeared yellow hospital gown for better access as I stepped forward to do compressions in his stead. On tiptoes, I clasped my right hand on top of my left and bore the heel of my hand into her sternum, to the beat of "Another One Bites the Dust," the song they'd told us in CPR training has 100 beats per minute. My fingers splayed over her breast, and I couldn't help noticing how soft her skin was. It felt like baby powder made solid. I didn't stare at her face, because I knew it would worsen the nausea I was already feeling. The smell of bile filled the room, and there was no mistaking the sickness in it. I stood on tiptoes to be right above her, focusing on the placement of my hands as I pushed and released. I knew the heart needed to both compress and relax in order to pump blood and fill back up. After a minute, I was already tiring and feeling a little light-headed, but every shift was supposed to be two minutes. I kept going, focusing on doing everything I could to try to save this life that didn't seem inclined to be saved.

Crack. I felt it under my hands and paused in terror.

"Keep going," my attending said. "It's okay."

I had broken one of her ribs, or maybe even her sternum . . . I kept going, knowing that breaking ribs is a very common occurrence in CPR, and that people can still be resuscitated even with broken ribs. I kept jack-hammering as best as I could, mortified at what had just happened. I had physically broken a dead woman's bones . . .

"It's been two minutes," Ken said.

"Okay, switch in now," I said, quickly backing against the window a couple feet away. I was nauseous, light-headed, exhausted, terrified, but resolved to do everything I could to help. I wanted to do my best in this room. I wanted to be a part of the process of making sure everything had been done to save this woman, because that's what she had wanted. Every patient who comes into the hospital is asked if they would want CPR or not, and is educated on what that means. She too, had been asked, and she wanted every chance she could get to continue living. So here we were, trying. But it wasn't looking good. She had pulled out her IV line a half hour before breathing in all the bile that stopped her heart. Part of CPR is administering adrenaline into the patient's veins to stimulate her heart. Without an IV, the attending physician was trying to puncture a vein in her fragile skin while we were doing chest compressions. He wasn't able to find one, and so the next step was drilling a hole into her shin to then push a needle in and get the adrenaline into her bloodstream through her bone marrow. When they did that, the skin around her bone puffed up instead; the adrenaline had leaked right back out of her bone into the surrounding tissue rather than going up to her heart. They drilled a second hole further up, and when they shot the adrenaline in there, it came back out the previous hole. They covered the lower hole up and shot more in, doing everything they could, but it wasn't looking good.

"Her feet are cold," someone said.

It was my turn to switch back in, and I could feel the tension in my calves as I tiptoed up to position myself.

"Boomp, boomp, boomp . . . another one bites the dust . . ."

This time, I realized how insanely warped it was to be singing that song in my head. The callousness of the CPR instructors hadn't seemed that big of a deal when I was learning it, but now it sure did. An alternative song with the same beat was "Stayin' Alive," so I switched to that, willing the lyrics into my hands and silently apologizing to this woman. I didn't think there was really any chance of her coming back to this life, but I wanted her to have every chance, and I intended to give her every good intention and well-executed compression that I could.

"We'll go for one more round of compressions and then call it," my attending said. I switched back out, heaving air into my own lungs and feeling my heart beating fast. If she had half the amount of those two functions, she'd be able to survive. But she was still ashen, with no muscle tone to speak of, lying there being pounded on and stabbed, because this is what she had wanted. We'd been going for about twenty-five minutes, and there had been no change, except for the extensive physical damage we had inflicted. I wondered if she really knew what she had asked for. Did she really want to stay alive, only to continue being sick? Had it been a fear of dying? A fear of leaving her children on their own? Was she following an expectation to always exhaust all options before admitting defeat, even if that meant losing parts of yourself in the process?

"Stop compressions," Dr. Rudis said. He felt for her carotid arteries, and then said, "Time of death, 6:57 a.m." A nurse reported it, and the noises were now slow and muffled, in stark contrast to the frenzied futility of the last twenty-seven minutes. I was grateful to the nurse who said, "Let's clean her up," because it felt like an apology to help straighten the blankets over her and wipe off some of the bile from her chest. I wanted to apologize for my part in the trauma we just put her through, to convey my condolences for our failure to keep her alive when she had wanted us to.

As I left the room, trying to put my head back together to present all of the new patients we admitted overnight to the team taking over from us, I couldn't help despairing a little over my worry that society isn't able to welcome death calmly. Puking up your stomach and getting ribs broken and bones pierced, all while lying naked in a room of strangers isn't peaceful. It isn't dignified. It's a gruesome tool that isn't used as rarely as it can actually work.

I walked back up the stairs, my shirt drenched in sweat, the smell of bile filling my nostrils, and made a note to think later about the philosophy of death. For now, it was all I could do to make it up the stairs in my sleep-deprived, terrified exhaustion.

IANNA H-M. | United States

We Are Not That Different, You and Me

I stand there pondering whether this is an exercise in mob mentality. None of us—except perhaps the few eager surgeons-to-be—would ever dream of slicing up a human body by ourselves. Yet now, armed with scrubs and scalpels, all acting in unison, this was somehow acceptable. I have no special interest in the surgical specialties, but I know that this is a rite of passage and I try to accept it as such. "A tremendous opportunity," I continue to soothe myself. "Yet another way to access the information you will need to care for patients."

I do indeed enjoy anatomy. I enjoy the subject matter, the hours I spend looking at textbooks, memorizing nerve innervations and muscle origins, but it is the actual physical act of dissecting that leaves me a little uneasy. Nonetheless, I tell myself to gird my loins and give my best attempt. Our first task is to flip the cadaver on its back, to begin the dissection on the posterior surface. The term, "dead weight," takes on tangible meaning. My brain begs for a moment to think—a moment to process this. *You feel fine right now, but how will you feel when you're alone at night in your apartment? What are you doing? What have you done?* I am the third in my group of five to dissect. The first point of contact makes everything seem even more real. I almost feel my cadaver's presence floating above me, encouraging: *It's okay. My time on earth is done. This is your journey.* I arm my scalpel with its blade. Then there is blood all over my hands. Something is wrong. I look to where the blade has lodged itself in my arm. Someone yells that the cut might be deep. Another voice bellows . . . something about the school infirmary. *What is happening to you?*

It is ten minutes later. I find myself lying supine on an exam table, being prepped and disinfected—being made ready to be cut into. The person doing the prepping makes light-hearted jokes to calm me. I am scared. I am alone. The jokes do not calm me. Yet the person continues. I hear the rain outside and my mind drifts to her, her on the icy table, her who I had named Nancy. The instructor's words echo in my mind, Treat with respect! She was loved!

The joker is still talking. My mind drifts again. I am on a table just like her, ready to be cut into. I whisper, *Treat with respect. She is loved.*

NARA M. | United States

TWO

SOJOURNER

> To wake up each morning to a new day, unsure of
> what it will bring, and to ease into this day's flow,
> with gratitude for whichever turn it takes.
> *Katherine F.*

The pursuit of dreams often leads us far beyond comfort and country. We leave our homes to lands near and far to start medical school or residency, and while there, repeatedly uproot ourselves as we move between rotations or interviews. The reflections in this chapter touch on trainees' journeys of discovery in medicine—how they navigate new terrains within and without, and find their spaces in medicine.

Five Thousand Miles

You've traveled far
To learn to care;
For friends, maybe,
But for strangers, likely.
Hopefully someone's done the same too;

So that when you need it,
Someone will show up—
Friend or stranger—
With a degree in you.

TOLU K. | United States

Physician: Healer and Historian

An American poet and political activist, Muriel Rukeyser, said the universe is made of stories, not of atoms. I believe her.

I walked gingerly into the adult emergency services for my first shift as a volunteer at a legendary New York City public hospital. I sported a crisply ironed red polo with "Emergency Department Volunteer" embroidered in white stitch.

As a seasoned story writer and storyteller, I had armed myself with a pocket notebook, and a pen, to tie up my hair. I was both ambivalent and apprehensive to perform alongside my colleagues, who were focused pre-medical students in rapacious pursuit of the coveted MD degree. My instrument of choice was a writing utensil, so it was with good reason I shivered at the thought of nearing a stethoscope or a scalpel. Suffering from an incurable case of imposter syndrome, I feared someone would detect that I was better at languages than logarithms. *Qu'est-ce que c'est organic chemistry?*

I feared for my life and for the life of the patients I was about to meet. I wondered how I, a hesitant traveler on a circuitous path to a healthcare career, managed to get myself into a prestigious summer program and into the hustle and bustle of one of the nation's busiest emergency departments (EDs). To the house staff, I thought, I could contribute nothing more than open-mindedness, keen curiosity, and readiness to learn. To the patients, I could contribute nothing more than an attentive ear and hearty conversation. But over the ten weeks of the summer program, as I observed the importance of communication in medicine, I learned that the skills I sharpened as a writer are invaluable assets to the medical profession. While the rest of my cohort was drawn to peeking through closed curtains at strangers' open fractures, I was more interested in observing the beautiful, intimate relationship between doctor and patient.

A good physician hears a chief complaint. A great physician listens, absorbs, and interprets the story of illness. I was awestruck at the divide, the marked difference between the physicians who seemed to connect easily with patients and those who did not. While some physicians overlooked a basic introduction, others showed their mastery of the art of medicine by nourishing human connection. While some physicians sifted through medical charts for past medical histories and chief complaints, others read symptoms through body language or subtle gestures.

I took careful note. I penned my discoveries in the lines of my notebook, constantly editing my pro/con list that detailed why I wanted, and didn't want, to become a doctor. I admired the personable interactions physicians shared with unfamiliar people and longed for the same. But with each interaction, I noticed that there was a dire, perhaps a severely underestimated, need for narrators in medicine.

As a volunteer, I befriended strangers. The interviewer in me asked unscripted questions. I comforted distraught patients and created strong bonds of trust. I was graciously welcomed into patients' lives. They let me trade sandwiches for their life stories. They confided in me their stories of love and loss, desire and death, melancholy and madness. I ended that summer with a strong sense of accomplishment, purpose, and gratitude. I learned that even as a native storyteller, I could be a healer. I could use my skill as a writer for the greater good of humanity. I learned that like the universe, medicine is indeed made of stories, not of atoms.

My experience as an ER volunteer confirmed the value of narrative competence in medical practice. For instance, residents were critiqued on how well they shared patient stories with attendings during rounds. Additionally, physicians concisely inscribed their patients' stories in charts. These observations, among others, made clear that the physician's story intertwines with the patient's. At the bedside, these stories overlap and weave together to build a special, shared narrative. Like a text, the physician closely reads the patient's body, with the patient as the character, illness as the conflict, and treatment plan as the resolution. Simply put, the physician is both healer and historian. The practice of medicine is a tactful balance, a constant challenge to distill information rapidly and responsibly. Physicians, like writers, read between the lines, they interpret unspoken words to make a diagnosis and propose treatment. In this way, a physician is both writer and editor of a life story.

SONAL K. | United States

A version of this piece was originally published on *the Almost Doctor's Channel.*

The Journey That is Third Year

I'm now three-quarters through the most unscripted year of my medical education. This is the year my classmates and I transition from the classrooms to the hospitals, where we rotate through highly specialized clinical settings. After each of these sequential mini-experiences, one hopes to have learned distinct styles of clinical decision-making, while getting a sense of the overall flow of patient care. However, the timing and source of this education is typically unpredictable.

This is a very personal year for us, as one student's experiences can differ markedly from another's. Geographically, we are dispersed over three tertiary care hospitals, divided into several major clinical departments at different times of the year, distributed over multiple specialty clinics, stretching from the main hospitals to suburban commutes, and evaluated by a medley of physicians and residents with distinct personalities and professional styles. The educational uncertainties abound.

I started the year off with a lot of enthusiasm and a hint of desperation; I wanted to get the fullest sense of clinical care, knowing that I might never again experience many of these clinical settings. Adding to my energy was the expectation that our clinical roles would be ill-defined. Wanting to immerse myself in new hands-on experiences, I got involved in any clinical opportunity that came my way.

NOVELTY AND BEWILDERMENT

Some of these experiences have been really unsettling. In my first month, I eagerly rushed to multiple traumas in the emergency department. In my first such encounter, a woman who had been struck by a high-speed van frantically began tugging at my scrubs as my team assessed her, en route to the CT scanner—with multiple pelvic fractures and heavy abdominal bleeding, she died only a few hours later. I had so many questions, and I could not fully grasp why things happened as they did. That same week, I performed chest compressions to help resuscitate a dying man—at one dramatic point, he nearly lifted his chest straight at me, only to die minutes later. Again, the team's thought process and expectations were unclear to me.

The heightened intensity of these experiences, mixed with their novelty and my bewilderment, is only part of what makes the third year of medical school a difficult transition. The other challenge is in figuring out what to take away from these strange experiences, what to learn.

Much of this year's learning is self-propelled by brazen confidence, and often only restrained by situational awareness and a sense of propriety. Getting involved has its risks, but my pursuit of a fuller education always begs for more.

After seeing a few trauma cases on the late night of my second twenty-four hour call, I asked a friendly Emergency Department resident to teach me and my co-medical student how to use the ultrasound machine. The next day, I rolled the machine into a mild-looking trauma evaluation and quickly started the mandatory ultrasound exam of the patient's abdomen. Having successfully completed three-quarters of the exam, I then had to confess that I was too inexperienced to finish the cardiac portion of the test. The resident across from me did not mind, and took over from where I left off. Although I felt like I might have intruded on professional patient care, I left feeling somewhat emboldened.

However, such enthusiasm has been tempered by less desirable clinical encounters. The most frightening case happened as I was instructed to depress and elevate a device to manipulate the uterus during a laparoscopic hysterectomy. While doing so, I accidentally perforated the patient's posterior vaginal wall. After making note of the incident to my team and then guiltily watching the repair, I had one of the worst feelings of my third year. Luckily, the clinical fellow, Dr. A.R., had the sensitivity and generosity to reassure me that it was not my fault, that the patient's tissue was unusually thinned.

In another personal catastrophe on the wards, I had just learned how to draw blood from a patient's radial artery, and with the permission of my resident, decided to try it myself. My thoughts clouded by the small victory of a successful arterial blood draw, I didn't realize I had incorrectly capped the tube. A moment later, I showered the patient's blood all over myself and the sub-intern.

Experiences like these have been humbling. A lot can be said about self-driven learning, but the opportunity for making mistakes is equally frightening or inhibiting. So the question remained, how and where can I safely gain further clinical experience and education?

THE HIDDEN FACULTY

Outside of a few specialized weekly lectures, most of the learning is on-the-job. Some faculty describe this as a "hidden curriculum," but the unpredictable or unreliable nature of this education makes me hesitate to call it a curriculum. Some attending physicians and residents were more involved than others. And many, though not all, patients were receptive to being cared for by students.

Fortunately, in the medical profession, there are individuals at all levels willing to support and foster a junior trainee's advancement. If there is such a thing as a hidden curriculum, then these special individuals are the hidden faculty. So, I kept track of my clinical heroes—those doctors and patients who have inspired me during the year.

MY HEROES

While rotating at a pain management clinic, I encountered a scenario where one doctor's thoughtful clinical reasoning spared a patient from an unnecessary and invasive spinal procedure. Rather than let his residents practice the more complicated procedure, he directed a simpler study to assess other causes of the patient's back pain. Following a puncture with an X-ray guided needle, the patient tearfully exclaimed "that's it [the pain], right there!" These tears were partly due to a painful sacro-iliac joint, but mostly to the relief of finally having a diagnosis for her mysterious back pain.

Highly qualified residents, too, stand out on my list of clinical heroes. There's Dr. R.P., a force of incredible optimism and motivation. Beloved by her colleagues and students, she personified some of the best qualities in a resident and a team player. There's Dr. N.S., who was an incredible joy to work with, and taught me much about compassionate and often multi-lingual patient care. There's Dr. E.C., who stood out for consistently following through with his offers to review my presentations before patient-centered pediatrics rounds. There's Dr. R.V., a male resident who thoughtfully walked me through the delicate task of performing my first pelvic exams. And then there's Dr. P.C., who gave me unprecedented responsibility late one night, to assist on an emergent surgical evacuation of a brain bleed in a rapidly deteriorating patient.

Equally important are the distinct patients who have taught or inspired my clinical education this year. These patients typically had a delightful mix of optimism and emotional connectedness, despite their illnesses. I often think of an elegant, elderly patient who sang an Irish melody as she was carted into the OR for gallbladder surgery. Or the memory of a delightful young patient standing and laughing with friends only hours after the successful resection of her brain tumor. Or my bedside experience with Mr. L, considered a clinical burden by my team, but who shared his resilience and personal strength with me, including sharing his audio recordings that he made at home, while he was plugged in to multiple catheters, bags of fluid, and other electronic equipment. Then there are my multiple patients who patiently let me practice interviewing them in Spanish, my third language.

Lastly, this year has been marked by an intersection of professional and highly personal growth. I started my third year only days after my wife and I got married. Because she was midway through residency training, she had accumulated many experiences with which I could not yet relate. However, my wife and I now share more of each other's experiences, and she has been a major contributor to my perspectives on residency and training. Given the challenges clinical responsibilities can place on any relationship, our new intellectual bonds have been an unexpected benefit.

GIVE AND TAKE

As I think about my third-year education, I can't help but notice how I have been led towards more serious mentorship roles. Soon after starting this year, I began a longitudinal primary care experience at a student-run clinic in Chelsea. At this clinic, I am referred to as a "senior clinician," and am expected to not only see patients, but also mentor a junior trainee in the second year of medical or nursing school.

I was a reluctant teacher at first. Lacking confidence about my own knowledge base coming out of my PhD, I was surprised to have things to offer my junior colleagues. However, my teaching skills improved over the year. As I learned more about the gaps in my education, I began to find ways to improve my junior students' clinical experiences: choosing teaching topics, giving pointers on history taking, demonstrating the use of an ophthalmoscope, and giving presentation tips.

In summary, this year has been incredibly challenging year, strengthened by hidden faculty: specific physicians, residents, and patients. In so many ways, I hear the wheels turning in the cycle of professional training. As I get further in my training and take whatever I can receive, I also see how I might be called upon to give back.

CAMERON S. | United States

A Year of Firsts

San Francisco and its curmudgeon Karl
presented faces of old pen pals and high school gals.
The comfort of lingering love keeps possibilities alive,

but the first lesson was naught for complacency;
stand strong with the tide.

This newfound clarity returned to eastern shores;
Soon questioned by feelings of un-want from those forced
    through hospital doors.
I learned to sit, listen, and practice empathy;
With time we waded through waves with trust, so worthy.

Autumn brought new hope of imprinting on a specialty;
A birthday well spent in a stressful delivery.
But what I found in the end was unexpected and ironic,
the presence of a midwife, a mirage of calming magic.

A youngin' in years with bright eyes to show,
I glowed with each fourteen-hour work day, no room for groans.
Defining passion in one moment alone,
I shed a sea of tears when the adrenaline dissipated,
a warrior dethroned.

Even my nomadic soul knows a home,
no surprise that I was again ready to roam.
Teetering on this bridge of transience taught me:
Sail away not for escape but for the next chapter of your story.

Hurry up then halt time, with gods of nature I conferred.
On the beach with horses, on the ocean with otters,
I was undeterred.
Nurture rebellion, plant seeds of gratitude,
I finally found my haven to cultivate solitude.

Glorified visions of the simple life:
A farmer, a fisherman, live off the land without regard for the
    strife
of school and residency, but the heartache of sacrifice

showed me that medicine is indeed my calling. So for the firsts of this year, let's cheer thrice.

LYE-YENG W. | United States

Milk, Milk, Milk

I am in Calcutta, India—a lifetime ago. I have just finished several months working as a doctor in a rural village in the south, taking some time before residency, and it is time to head home. Before I leave India, I stuff a backpack with my worldly possessions and hit the trail. I am a pilgrim, of sorts, at the beginning of my career, wondering where my life will lead. I go to Calcutta. I seek the home of Mother Teresa.

After a thirty-hour, bone-crunching ride up the east coast, the train disgorges me into the swamp, the fantastic energy of Calcutta—the morass of tuk tuk wallahs, the languid dust and wheezing heat, the stench of gasoline and spices. It is great. Calcutta is a city of pilgrims and refugees from the surrounding villages. Everyone is hustling, looking for something. I am merely one more.

I hitch a ride over the Howrah bridge and stash my backpack in a hostel. I open my guidebook and take to the streets—a refugee in search of refuge. The refuge I seek is, of course, the Mother House of Mother Teresa. I am captivated by this woman who modeled sacrifice and love. I want to stand in the doorway of the Mother House, where her ministry began.

She had died a few months before and I wanted to stand in the cloud of her powerful memory, absorb her somehow, become more like her. I walk where she walked, down the narrow streets, guide-book open to the map, past the stands selling jasmine and turmeric, a mother bathing her child on the sidewalk, a man fixing a clock, holding it between his feet.

I am closer now, closer, nearly at the dot marked "Mother House" on my map. I walk past a motorcycle fix-it shop, a gray two-story warehouse, the local chapter of the Indian Communist Party, a bread store, and then I am nowhere. I am on a bridge at a busy intersection. I have passed Mother Teresa's House. I missed it somehow.

From the corner of my eye, I see two nuns fly out of the alleyway next to the gray warehouse. I backtrack and look up to see a simple, bronze plaque on the wall, green with age—"Missionaries of Charity." The Palace for Mother Teresa's Empire of Compassion is a two story, gray warehouse. In my heart, I expected something more—something more gothic? More Disney? But really, a refitted warehouse makes perfect sense. She was a woman who traded her Nobel Prize dinner for rice and beans for the poor.

I stand before this weathered brass sign, this dilapidated building, taking it all in. I feel a tug on my wrist. Before me is a thin girl, maybe twelve years old. She wears a blue dress, a little worn, but clean. She has a twisted right hip and a spastic arm. I brace myself, for she is the one millionth person to ask me for money that day.

"What is your name?" she asks. She is cheerful and friendly, and addresses me as if we were at a church barbecue.

"I am Ben. What is your name?"

"I am Molly. Buy me some milk. Milk. Milk. Milk." Not a request. A command.

In the shadow of Mother Theresa's home, how could I say no? I follow Molly as she limps to the grocer. "Milk. Milk. Milk," she commands.

The grocer places a large box of instant dry milk on the counter.

"How much?" I ask.

"300 Rupees," he says.

I balk. "300 rupees?" That is almost ten American dollars, and more than I spend on food in a week on the road. I do some math. I have just over eighty dollars-worth of rupees, and five more days of travel. It would be very tight indeed.

"Milk. Milk. Milk," smiles Molly.

"300 Rupees! Too expensive!"

"Milk. Milk. Milk."

"No Milk! No Milk! No Milk!" Perhaps I am too tired, too cheap, too rational, too beaten down by the trail. The flood of excuses and rationalizations tastes like bile, but I do not yield. "What good will this do for her in the long run?" I think to myself. But this time, in the shadow of Mother Teresa's memory, it is different.

I hesitate. I doubt. And the moment is over before I can change my mind. Molly looks at me. She smiles — no judgment, no regret. She gives me the sweetest, most joyful smile as if she knows something that I do not. She turns and melts into the crowd. She is gone. The angel with the twisted hip disappears. I am left with the taste of bile and regret. Milk. Milk. Milk.

The money in my pocket is moist with sweat, practically dissolving in the Calcutta heat. I saved 300 rupees. But at what cost?

BENJAMIN D. | United States

Secret Languages

When my mother was upset, or when she was very happily surrounded by her sisters, her words would switch to Javanese, a fluent, secret language her mind opted to use in extremes of emotion. I lived in Jakarta rather than my mother's hometown of Surakarta, and so I learned Bahasa Indonesia first, but picked up some Javanese words to learn to be on my mother's good side, and to eavesdrop on my aunties' conversations. Unlike my mother's family, my father's older siblings went to a Dutch school and, consequently, learned to speak Dutch. At the dining table, the air ringing with the chatter of rickshaws and buzzing of mosquitoes, they spoke in hushed, guttural tones to mask certain details I would never know. Between the two Dutch- and Javanese-speaking camps, my older sister and I felt frequently left in the dark.

When we finally moved to New York, the fast, wide-voweled American English that my third-grade classmates used, peppered with "likes" and "ums," exhausted me. Yet, my sister and I vowed to never speak Bahasa Indonesia at home, hoping to lose our accents and blend in. Ironically, many years later, when our identities became hyphenated and our passports privileged, we took safety again in speaking in Bahasa Indonesia, so that others could not understand what we said, and then in Spanish, so our parents could not understand.

It never dawned on me that any of the languages I had mastered could still be spoken in a way that would exclude me. But in medicine, I found that people spoke a form of English I had never come across:

> Patient is a [insert age], with significant PMHX of this that and the other, coming in for [insert CC]. Blah blah H&P, ROS, medications bid, tid, qd, wait, now daily, allergies, family hx of DM, CHF, CAD, HTN, physical exam with AVSS, NAD, CV of RRR, Pulm of CTAB, Abd NTTP, skin warm, pink, cap refill brisk, one liner of all above information gathered with assessment, plan of vanc-zosyn, OOB, consult PT and OT.

As medical students, like my sister and I were, we are often left in the dark. On the first day of my clinical year, I remember being barraged by abbreviations with meanings I could neither imagine nor know. I would give presentations with complete information, but the different order in which I placed them reduced me to inept, resulting in poor evaluations, not for the lack of knowledge, but for the lack of conformity. In medicine, I found that language clearly delineated the hierarchy of education, highlighted the letters lacking at the end of my name, and emphasized power structures rivaling those of empires.

I was most befuddled in and around death. When I encountered my first two deaths on my first rotation, I jotted words on paper, not to help me understand, but to try to capture how fleeting life can be, as cliché as it is true. The words were my last memories of the patients and the events surrounding their deaths. I could sense worry in people's tones and in their actions, but worry was almost immediately followed by a sense of hurry, on to the next patient. The word "death," surprisingly, was never mentioned.

> **We lost —**
> *can I just go home? —patient*
> *just an episode of hypotension.*
> *I don't know what to do. —intern*
> *she was a demented woman. agitated achy cold.*
> *you are just going to leave? —family*
> *stay away from that room. aggressive family.*
> *in and out.*
> *beat and stop.*
> **—Two.**

Like I had in my first years in the United States, again I found myself trying to assimilate and conform, eager to lose my previous layperson speak for the native white-coat tongue. However, this time, unlike my experience as an eight-year-old, I was not certain I wanted to fully join this new culture, because it likely meant losing a large part of myself, how I had learned to communicate in the world, to be in the world.

Thus far, I have learned that language gives you power: power to communicate, power to open an unknown world, and to close it, power to exclude. As I have gained mastery of medical lingo, I too have begun to use words in ways that exclude certain listeners and opacify information: on family-centered rounds, I slip into jargon only the medical team might understand; in a patient's postoperative report, I dismiss his pain, noting it "as expected." This has not been a conscious process, but rather one resulting from immense pressure, both externally and within, to fit in. As I rise in the ranks of the hospital's hierarchy, I feel myself becoming sturdier with knowledge, but somehow farther from connection. I acknowledge that this is part of the learning process. I am supposed struggle to learn medical jargon, practice with it, and perhaps get carried away while giving oral presentations on rounds. I know I will yet learn how to both use proper medical terms *and* include everyone in the room, whether medical professional or layperson. But I want to own up to my failings along the way. I want to stay conscious and aware of when I slip, to continue to find balance between knowledge and connection.

As I enter into residency, I long to be fluent in the medical language and simultaneously rediscover my former self again, the self that lived in a world where it was blasphemous not to understand a patient's illness in the context of her life outside the hospital. Acknowledging that acquiring a new language, a new power, *can* be used to open doors, rather than exclude, I long to be fluent in the medical language to fully connect with patients again.

If I were to start clinical years—or really, medical school—all over again, I would ask myself, "Who are you and what are your values?" I'd write my answers down and instruct my brain to remember what I had written, so that the process of assimilation would not mean the losing of my humanity and sense of self.

VANESSA S. | United States

THREE

ISLANDS, AND THE BRIDGES BETWEEN

> I'm so spacey at family dinner . . . just mentally
> reviewing which antimicrobials bind to which
> bacterial ribosomal subunits.
> I used to be present.
>
> *Anonymous*

*Medical trainees choose medicine for various reasons. Often,
loved ones play key roles in moving us towards medicine, and
perhaps, away from it too. The reflections in this chapter highlight
the many ways in which our dreams are often not ours alone.
The reflections also speak to how the connections we make
in medicine overcome the isolation that medical training often
brews.*

To Flames, and Those That Fan Them

As a young boy, Car Wash Saturdays were something of a
household tradition. Every so often, on a Saturday, my dad would
take the car to the wash and my older brother and I would go
along. On one of these Saturdays when I was five, I remember

pretending to feed my father and older brother medicine—juice, really—out of a spoon while we waited at the car wash. A few weeks before, I had gone with my aunt to work. She worked as a receptionist to a doctor, now probably old and grey. Save for the sore injection sites on my small shoulders after periodic vaccination visits, I knew nothing about what being a doctor entailed. But I was intrigued by this man in a white coat: what exactly was it that he did after he ushered his patients in to his office and closed the door?

Fourteen years later, on the first day of medical school, I realized that I still didn't really know what being a doctor entailed. If I was honest, most of my impressions about medicine had been shaped by what I had seen on *Grey's Anatomy* or *House*. But I was proud that a dream that had taken root in a five-year-old's heart following a chance encounter with a man in a white coat was coming to fruition. I might not have known what I was signing up for exactly, but I knew I was finally going to find out what lay behind that man's door of endless possibilities. I was finally going to be the man in the white coat.

As my journey through medical school has progressed, it has struck me how our dreams often aren't fully ours. Many people have played one part or another in sparking flames or keeping them alive. My granny, for instance, spent most of her life in apartheid South Africa, and as a black female that meant she couldn't dream of being more than a domestic worker or sales assistant at a store. So, once I voiced my interest in medicine to her at five, my dream became hers. "Ntinga ntakandini uyonqandwa ziinkwenkwezi," she said once in our native isiXhosa. *Aim for the stars so that if you do fall, you fall to the tops of the highest trees.* Her words have served as sources of inspiration and motivation in trying times. Recently, she got to see me assist a family member who had had an asthmatic episode. I am glad that in small ways, she is getting glimpses into this dream that is partly hers.

Now halfway through my degree, I can say I know a lot more about what being a doctor entails and thankfully, I like what

I have seen so far. Medicine continues to be a lesson in self-discovery, difficult but rewarding. As I delve further into what lies behind my own door, I imagine that my five-year-old self is proud that his dream is taking root.

MBULELO K. | South Africa

History-Taking Tips from Grandma

I learned how to take a proper medical history from my grandmother. Ralph, the shy boy who lived across the street from me, came over one day to teach me how to rollerblade. Within moments of ringing the doorbell, my grandmother greeted him with a cup of Assam tea in one hand, and Mauritian treats in the other. In her wobbly English, she started with her innocent probing: "Have you eaten? Which house did you say you live?" I witnessed Ralph, the silent ninth-grader who had a monochromatic emotional repertoire, open up and start to talk. By the end of the conversation, Ralph and my grandmother had shared a meal, giggled together over his big sister's bad cooking, and reminisced about their experiences at their immigration ceremonies. Leave it up to my grandmother to unveil your hobbies, family history, and recreational drug use all before you take off your coat.

When my grandparents got married, they opened a small store that sold groceries and baked goods. Being a storekeeper required remarkable interpersonal skills, and from the thugs of Rosehill to the housewives of Port Louis, my grandma knew how to talk to literally anyone. She connected with people just by virtue of being interested in who they were. She was charming and street smart and knew how to deescalate a situation when clients were unhappy or disappointed. She always made people feel at home and listened to. My grandma never learned these skills from a textbook; they were unspoken lessons drawn from her everyday interactions that required kindness and empathy.

For me, on other hand, getting people to open up has always been challenging. As a first-year medical student, I frequently found myself turning to my clinical skills handbook for help. "Ask open ended questions," it said. So I would sit down beside the patient at eye level (so as not to be intimidating), smile at "appropriate" times, and nod at the correct frequency. When I spoke to patients, it was with the hyperawareness of a self-conscious dancer. I always felt like I was performing (think Ashlee Simpson and her lip-syncing disaster). Intense awkwardness pervaded my clinical encounters and made connecting with patients impossible. But after visiting my grandma after my first year of medical school, I realized that much of what I had learned in my clinical classes were basic life skills that people, like my grandma, intuitively knew just by virtue of listening, caring, and being attentive to the needs of those around them.

My grandmother never went further than elementary school education, yet her ability to make people comfortable enough to divulge their life histories would impress even experienced physicians. I hope that in the future, I can embody what my grandmother always knew intuitively: that you only need to invite people to sit down, ask if they have eaten, and let them tell you where they have been, where they plan to go, and what you can do to help them on their journey.

STEPHANIE W. | Canada

Letter to Wanita Armstrong

Dear Wanita,

When I began writing this, Sue had just informed me of your passing. Just over a week before she did, I remember visiting

New Hampshire for an exam. As Sue knows, visiting you one last time was a top priority. I remember tucking your hand underneath your blanket, talking with Sue for half an hour, and worrying whether your grimaces were from pain. Sue had nonchalantly asked for a phone number by which to contact me. "There's no rule book on how to feel at this point," I had said to Sue that day outside your room, listening to your slow, labored breathing.

Weeks later, when Sue informed me of your passing, a shower of memories shook me as I processed the information. During that last visit, I remember sitting in my car after saying goodbye, and feeling how real and palpable the care and love was in your room, in that house, in your last days and months when I got to know you:

I remember turning into Sue's driveway, balancing a hot C&A's pizza (with onions, peppers, mushrooms, olives, and extra sauce, just how you like it) on one palm and your diet Pepsi with my Bayada volunteer nametag on the other, the crunch of snow new to me because I had been in California the entire winter. I remember smiling at your first bite, and smiling when you furtively glanced my way when the toppings fell off your fork.

I remember the silence we shared in your room as I sat next to you, when your eyelids were heavy and drooping. After a few minutes, I would wake you up by asking about the blue jays you saw every morning eating birdseed out of the window. You would recollect about the bleeding heart plants outside your Norwich residence, which grew uncontrollably in your garden. I remember reading the *Valley News* to you when we could no longer play cribbage, talking about the Lebanon church that burned down, and, as you would say, "the horrible man" that beat your beloved Hilary. I would always tell you, "No more falling, Wanita!" and you would say "oookayy, I won't . . ."

I remember knocking and immediately opening the door of your Norwich home, knowing that you wanted me to come in; to an outsider, it probably looked like I was breaking into your home. I would habitually grab your cribbage board before you tried to tell me where it was "this time" (which was where I left it). Even though you taught me how to play, I never had the courage to tell you that we weren't actually keeping score correctly; or that when our games were really close, I knew when you would take a few extra spaces with your peg and look to see if I had noticed. I wonder if you knew that I would move your own peg extra spaces, too, to see if you had noticed! I think the endearing look on your face when you would win that close game gave me more pleasure than it did you; but selfishly, I wasn't going to say anything.

Aside from those close games, for you, cribbage seemed less about playing than about reflecting—on the past, present, and an uncertain future. It was a surprisingly philosophical time. You would talk about your family's history in Norwich, your grand- and great grandchildren, the difficulties you faced as a mother, that Pat or Bob were going to visit that day, that Sue wanted you to live with her.

Throughout our time together, you showed by example how to be a good listener, and a kind friend. It is hard to know what it is like to be near death, facing life's decisions as your independence inevitably wanes. It is not something I think most adults think about: how to accept being dependent on others when you have been a beacon of strength and maternal care. You reinvented yourself, teaching me by example, and with such love and grace.

In my wallet I still have the photo you gave me of your ninetieth birthday, smiling brilliantly in your old chair. I don't think there is a better way to remember you.

No more falling, Wanita,

ANDREW H. | United States

No names have been changed. Published with family's permission.

Your Story Could Be Mine

You are telling me your story
All the things that you have done
The events you have experienced
The place where you come from

You are telling me your story
How you got where you are now
The ups and downs and twists and turns
Sometimes you aren't even sure how

You are telling me your story
And I see myself in you
I find myself starting to wonder
If that was me, what would I do?

"Walk a mile in my shoes" they say
"Trade places for a day"
How things could be so different
If I had grown up an alternate way

If I didn't have the tools I have
My supports in friends and family
Access to schools and medicines
Or the genetic protectors conferred to me

If I faced those same stressors you've experienced
Or a trauma when I was young
Would I have the resilience to cope with them
Or would I simply be overcome?

You are telling me your story
And these thoughts swirl around my head

Humbled before you, I sit
It could so easily be me in that chair instead

JENNIFER F. | United States

Listen to Empower

It was a particularly overcast day as I sat upon the radiator in my patient, Mr. C's room, holding his hand as he silently sobbed. I am not sure what led Mr. C to share his story with me, perhaps it was the weather—abnormally gloomy for July—or his uneasiness about his impending discharge. Regardless, I sat in silence processing the painful tale of addiction that resulted in his fourth admission. In that moment, I felt grateful that I had been granted the privilege of hearing the most intimate details of this man's life; that I had the education that allowed me to understand addiction as a disease; and that I had personal and professional experiences that nurtured my patience, compassion, and humility. As my mind began to drift, Mr. C's teary eye contact snapped me back into the moment. I searched for the words to offer support, understanding, and, most importantly, empowerment to change. "I'm rooting for you."

Throughout my first two years at Geisel, I (albeit, slowly) was able to gain a decent grasp on the pathophysiology behind the human body and disease. Yet, as my clinical years began, I realized that this offered only a superficial answer to the amorphous question of how people heal. The more patients I encountered, the more tangible the many barriers to health became. Whether my team was on the phone trying to get a pre-authorization from insurance or trying to develop a stable discharge plan for a homeless patient, we were never focused on merely the biological disease burden. Though I have always been an advocate for recognizing the social determinants of health, I soon realized that it isn't enough to just consider them. Whether you're like me, going into a field known for evaluating the "big picture," or not, who the patient is outside of the walls of the hospital must purposefully underlie every decision you make.

As you can imagine, this can be difficult. I watched many of my very capable and compassionate superiors walk into Mr. C's room, only to walk out condemning him to being "just another alcoholic" while quickly citing which tests and orders needed to be put in to stabilize and discharge him. It's not easy to look deeper while still keeping up with your endless clinical responsibilities. Yet, when I took my (much more abundant) time to hear Mr. C's story of abandonment and loss, it became so much easier to see him for who he was: a kind man in the throes of disease resulting from a lifetime of pain. Genuinely caring about him as an individual opened the door to so much more trust, and receptiveness to difficult conversations between Mr. C and his entire care team. Although this was his fourth admission, and all the same routine labs, tests, and evaluations were performed, his course also seemed to be following a new trajectory.

Mr. C exemplified to me how much of a disservice we do to patients by not hearing their stories or "big pictures." While stabilization of the acute issue is undeniably important, at the end of the day we are fooling ourselves if we think we are any of our patients' saviors. Our primary job should be to listen to our patients' stories in hopes of helping them regain control. This won't always be easy, but more often than not, it will be worth it. After all, I have found the most gratifying experiences not just in helping patients, but also in empowering patients to help themselves. Mr. C could not have said it better when we said goodbye the following day before his third stint in inpatient rehab, "Thank you for listening. I'm rooting for myself now, too."

TINA J. | United States

Intake

I chose to write down your words in red pen, to try to capture the color of your voice, the hue of your essence. I ask you to tell me more, in my effort to understand what I can. But I know I will still reduce your words to quickly (nervously) recited phrases and jargon, reducing you to the most compact, almost unrecognizable version of yourself. You tell me what hurts, you tell me your fears, you tell me you don't even know why you are telling me these things, your words dripping with mistrust and hope, inseparably intertwined. You shed a single tear, and I can't help but perseverate on its meaning, even two years later, almost to the day.

This tear could mean so many things, and I try to parse them out with you. Subtle nods, shrugged shoulders, inconspicuously contorted brows are the currency of safety I offer; anything I can possibly do to communicate support, security, interest. This tear, could it be the concentrated frustration of the seemingly endless line of case workers and police officers and interns—all strangers—walking or charging into the deepest part of your soul you'll allow? You've watched each one of us enter, then evaporate out of your space, leaving you to question if we were even there. I told you just minutes ago that I'm just another one of these characters making my brief debut. How many of us stop to consider the consequence of our intermittent interjection into someone else's world, someone else's pain?

This tear, could it be the slightest bit of fear skimmed from the top of your well of accumulated experiences? You tell me again you never talk about these things—it's not worth it—and I can see you trying to press it down once again. If only I could tell you that liquids are incompressible, tell you that I see your soul drowning through your eyes. This fear and pain are real, and I am momentarily distracted, wishing that you didn't feel like you had to carry this weight with you always, that there was a safe place for you to dispense it and give you reprieve. Or has the spout you use to dispense this liquid burden become rusted and clogged from years of favoring self-preservation over self-care?

I am still not sure what this tear means, two years later. I kept my promise to you: I haven't seen you again, because I'm really not so much different from those others that crash in and out of your life at their leisure. I kept my other promise too: I wouldn't forget your story. I still remember the sun rays bouncing off your umber skin, illuminating your ebony and sparsely-charcoaled curls, as you looked to the side and shrugged and maybe hoped that I missed the silent drop escaping the corner of your eye and tracing the curve of your cheek.

ALEXANDRA H-L. | United States

Bert

The first truly sick person I ever met was a forty-seven-year-old devoted husband and father of four named Bert. Noticing a slow increase in fatigue, he went to his PCP, who was concerned with this history and ordered, among other things, a CBC and fecal occult blood test (FOBT). Finding anemia and heme-positive stools, he scheduled Bert for a colonoscopy, which unfortunately found a mass in his right hemi-colon. A follow-up surgical excision with pathology confirmed the diagnosis of adenocarcinoma, and in conjunction with positron emission tomography-computed tomography (PET-CT), brought more dreaded news: the cancer had metastasized throughout his liver and into his lungs. Prognosis was grim: incurable, with an expected survival of twelve–eighteen months.

Fortunately, Bert beat the odds and remained alive eighteen months later. With a zest for life, he pursued all leads to beat back his disease while remaining focused on, and positive for, his family and friends. Traveling from Maine to Boston to New York City, he enrolled in two successive clinical trials, luckily receiving the experimental arms' chemotherapeutics in both. Still, these newer carcinotoxic cocktails only slowed his disease's toll, and by twenty-nine months, the downward trajectory was clear. At thirty-one months, surrounded by his wife and kids, he passed away.

You can probably tell that Bert was not a patient I met on the wards during a third-year clerkship. He was my dad. The experience of watching him take his last breath, and more importantly the thirty-one months leading up to it, was the seed that led me to medical school and the desire to fight disease. While long gone, as an intrinsic motivator, reminding me of why I'm here, I have frequently thought back to him these past two clinical years.

Why do I write about him? To hopefully remind you of your motivation for going through medical school. Focus on it to sustain you, and avoid getting swept up in fixating on the extrinsic evaluations that frequently do nothing but demean what brought you here. Nobody becomes a doctor to score well on evaluations and shelf exams. These are just cairns marking the trail up the mountain—important to reach and walk by, but not the reason for climbing. Resist becoming a cairn seeker. The true value of the process is that you're outside, gaining strength with each stride, and meeting and enriching the lives of Berts along the way.

ERIK A. | United States

Out of Silence, Into Medicine

"Are you a lesbian!?" Accusation and concern flew across the room at me as I walked into my house that afternoon. Recognizing a plea to calm their worries, my lips spat an immediate and convictive, "No! Of course not," like this idea had never crossed my mind. I saw from their faces that my answer had provided them the security they so desperately needed.

When I was younger, I loved to play Whack-a-Mole in arcades. In Whack-A-Mole, you hold a large mallet and run back and forth, trying to hit moles that pop out of their burrows. As you progress through the game, moles begin popping up faster and faster. It's impossible to guess where they will pop up next; it's like they can sense you, often surfacing furthest from your position. And then, the moles begin emerging two, three, four at a time, overwhelming you with a game-ending finish. Our minds are extraordinarily adept at keeping unwanted thoughts beneath the surface, preventing them from being acknowledged and consequently, becoming real. But thoughts, as they often do, come back, again and again, and at some point, you are forced to make a choice: you can fight them, containing and suffocating them, or you can make peace and let them surface as they please.

It was such a relief at first, to allow myself to privately claim the identity of "gay." But then my parents found out. There was confusion, yelling, destruction, broken relationships. "This has to be a phase." "You're too young to know what you want." "We are Catholic and now you will never get married or have children. Actually, please don't have children. It will be too hard for them." Being gay, or at least admitting to it, was an inconceivable idea to my parents. Their instinctual dismissal of my sexuality, though rooted in homophobia, was equally so in benevolence, meant to "protect me" and help steer me towards a happier and easier life.

While I credit my parents with so many of my individual strengths and successes, I will always carry scars from this acute, and chronic, rejection of my identity. During such a pivotal period of growth and psychological development, I was effectively muted at home. This experience, while difficult, has come to underlie my passion for hearing the stories of other silenced populations and has inspired my interest in social justice work. After coming out, I became more inquisitive about the world around me, examined my own family's intergenerational history of trauma, and became passionate about socioeconomic inequity and its intersection with health, reproductive justice, and gender-based violence. I came to view illness as the most fundamental manifestation of social injustices. From here, my path forward as a physician seemed almost undeniable.

It's challenging to think of a life filled with more human connection than that of a physician. As a medical student, I'm energized by patients and their unique narratives, narratives that inspire, change, and stay with you. Rotating through a range of specialties, often feeling lost, overwhelmed, and sleep deprived, I've often returned to the importance of individual narratives, and reminded myself of the privilege I have to be entering a profession that lets me elicit patient stories every day.

I'm excited to continue learning medicine and to cultivate my knowledge by carefully considering the perspectives and experiences of those often forgotten in the dominant pedagogical lens. As we listen to patients, it is important that we also refine our medical knowledge. After all, it is patient stories that give reason for our knowledge and theories to exist, change, and grow. We can only provide just healthcare when we listen carefully to patients, not only to their words, but also to their silences, which often speak volumes.

Being gay is an important part of my personal identity, but in a lot of ways, the process of coming out was so much more impactful in forming my sense of self and defining my core values. Coming out was transformative in my desire to understand difference, to empathize with human suffering, give voice to the voiceless, and in my ultimate decision to become a physician.

ASHLEY H. | United States

Oui, Je peux!

I studied medicine in Chad, and here, things lag. A degree that should take seven years takes ten. Tradition takes precedence over schooling: girls are to be found in the kitchen, not in classrooms or schools; medicine is reserved for men alone. So as I stood in my room, medical school diploma in hand, tears filled my eyes. It had been winding journey but I had made it to the other side.

I was fifteen and overflowing with dreams when my uncles had come with their proposition: *We have found a good husband for you. Every woman dreams of this and this is our duty to our late elder brother, your father. You're going to be happy in your new home.*

I was furious! They had no right. These same uncles had forced my two sisters out of school and into marriage: one sister had died in childbirth, the other was now divorced, with three children and limited prospects of returning to school. I had determined that my lot would be different, and so I refused. *Stubborn, Obstinate, Disrespectful to your father.* I was only seeking knowledge and autonomy, but with my refusal, I made enemies of my uncles.

Propelled by my desire to make more of my life, I worked hard to finish high school and afterwards, traveled to N'Djamena for university. It was difficult to leave my mother, but thankfully, my brother lived in N'Djamena and, in him, I found a father.

As I went through medical school, my brother took care of me and made sure I had what I needed. But soon enough, the need to be truly independent began to eat at me. This need spilled over into my medical training as I became increasingly eager to get into clinical care before the third year, when students typically got clinical exposure.

To satisfy my hunger for more, I chose to work in the bustling Emergency Room, an excellent place for hands-on learning. I had classes till about six p.m. every day, and then worked on the night service in the Emergency Room. My main task was learning to perform injections and offer first aid care on the medical and surgical services. The initial intent was to spend a week at a time on both services, but my thirst for learning was so strong that I often worked simultaneously on both services. The six months I spent in the ER proved quite rewarding, and

I was grateful to be taught by wonderful doctors, nurses, and senior medical students.

Next, I worked with a medical school teacher at a surgical clinic and in six months, was able to get certification to work, which also gave me extra money to send my mother gifts. Even though my brothers took care of everything she needed, I knew my mother liked gifts, and her calls to bless me for the gifts were precious to me. Encouraged by my family and as my school schedule got lighter, I took on more work and continued to send gifts home each month. (My mother was even able to spend a holiday with us in N'djamena!) I was happy. Things were wonderful and stable. Then one day, while I was at the clinic, my mom called, crying: *I don't want you to send me anything from today on! You refuse to get married! Most of the girls your age have three or four children! People here, and especially your uncles, are saying that you have become a prostitute, that's how you send me all these presents! That's beyond me and I can't bear to think of it!*

I was shocked. Me, a prostitute? Since when? So much time had passed, and I had accomplished so much, yet my uncles' mentalities still had not changed. But even more hurtful, they had managed to create a rift between my mother and me, so much so that she stopped taking my calls and outrightly refused to talk to me.

I have now reached the end of my medical school training. My last year was spent devoted to research and my thesis is now complete and brilliantly defended. Thankfully, my relationship with my mother, with much help from my brothers, has been restored. No one asks me any longer when I will marry. Maybe I'll get to it someday. But for now, I am focused on going back to my childhood home, to serve the province that raised me. I hope my presence signals to everyone that when a girl decides, she can do anything!

HABSITA A. | Chad

Ubuntu

Walk the road to success,
parents and teachers always address.
It will bring you great wealth;
Not just in cars and houses, but also in health.

But born with a heart of a gypsy,
this straight road leaves no room for mystery.
What of adventure and travel and love?
Away with the ten year plan, she said to the medicine gods
    above.

So off to Africa for a year
to make friends and get perspective, so clear.
She was attached to the independence of a single life;
Impervious to loneliness, fear or strife.

The best things in life are unexpected and free;
Good thing on principles and priorities they agree.
We make our own luck, don't leave it up to fate;
Where opportunity meets preparedness, they certainly relate.

Alas will she leave her heart in the city?
Or let the waves push her back and let it be.
With true love comes great responsibility;
And this ability to respond will form the roots of a sturdy tree.

LYE-YENG W. | United States

FOUR

SELF-DOUBT

My stomach has had a knot for 8 days.

Anonymous

Caring for patients is a heavy responsibility and medical trainees become even more aware of this as training progresses. Many become acquainted with the limitations of their minds and bodies and consequently, self-doubt becomes a steady companion. In this chapter, trainees reflect on their struggles with self-doubt—some reflections ask you to sit with the emotion, others provide you with glimpses of hope.

F is for Anatomy

I lost weight
from carrying your notes.
My back is hunched from nights
spent analyzing every curve in your frame.
Yet people say
I don't pay you much attention;
that I could do much better by you.

You know the truth,
yet are silent every time.
I broke up with her for you.
Do you even care?

GIDEON M. | Kenya

Knowing

"I don't know . . ."

My voice trailed off as I locked eyes with my supervisor's shoes. The panicked crack in my voice echoed down the hospital hallway, where we had both come to a standstill.

It was a Thursday afternoon, so naturally, my supervisor wore his Thursday shoes. Auburn. The laces had been forged into two perfectly symmetrical bows. The leather — as if the man had come straight from an airport terminal shoe-shiner — mirrored the fluorescent lights above us directly onto my face. I stood, helpless, in an inescapable spotlight of shame. The physician said nothing as we boarded the elevator down to the second floor. The weight of my disappointment, still, not enough to accelerate the sinking silo.

As we exited the elevator, my supervisor and I bid our farewell for the day. He didn't know my name, but his was one of grand reputation and esteem. My failure wore like a gold star on his white coat as he turned on his heels and floated towards the staff lounge. Tomorrow would be Friday. He would wear his Friday shoes.

Later that evening, I unraveled the doctor's question with a textbook acquired from the faculty library. Although it was far too late to undo my exposed inadequacy, I could not ignore the palpable gap in my knowledge. In medical school, filling my head with interminable material had become a daily test of endurance and purpose.

Medical culture's fixation on knowledge is appreciated by those we teach, and more so, by those we treat. Patients wait days, sometimes even months, for a glimmer of hope in understanding what ails them. Medical practitioners serve society as literal bodies of knowledge, fastened with the tools to heal and educate those who seek wisdom and guidance.

The irony of medicine is that we must know everything, and yet, we may never truly comprehend the patient experience. Where we see ourselves as the keepers of exclusive knowledge, our patients are the ones who ultimately carry its burden: the heartache of receiving a poor prognosis; the devastation of holding one's lifeless newborn; the dread of gripping a loved one's hand before a life-threatening operation.

So we must tread humbly and treat knowledge, not as a power to be wielded against those who do not possess it to the degree we do, but as a privilege, earned with time and experience. We must teach our learners this too, so that when they stand at the bedside, surrounded by questions and fear, both empathy and guidance can flourish.

And someday, armed with an audience of inquisitive medical students on an elevator ride down to the staff lounge, we must be sure to ask them one question . . .

Their names.

KAYLA S. | Canada

Time Within These Walls

> "Man created time and watches as his creation
> lords it over him."

My first watch was red. I remember, all too well, the heavy red face that showed the time in ones and twos, the black threaded strap that was often soaked with wrist sweat and that greeted my tongue with its salty taste whenever my hand came close enough to my face. My water-resistant watch followed me everywhere, a faithful companion on my right wrist. I was small, naïve, but with a superpower: I was in control of time. I was never late. Lateness was Mother's own doing. All I needed to do was to press a few buttons, watch the ones and twos become threes, fours, and zeros, and I had regained the time that Mum had lost. I was a god in my own right, unique and special. I may not have been the God that sent fire and brimstones, turned people to salt, or fed them sky bread like the one on Sunday, but I was god.

Growing up, and growing out of the idea that I was special, unique, or a god, wrenched pieces of me. Soon I realised that Mom was never late, I always was; that I could not regain time by pressing a few buttons on a watch. The real superhero was the woman that insulated me from the world and shielded me from realizing, too early, that I was not unique or special or a god, I was just me and that sometimes, that might not be enough.

Without sounding cliché, medical school is hard. Saying "not easy" would be an understatement, and saying that studying any course would be equally as hard is, well . . . I have had the privilege of attending one of Nigeria's prestigious medical schools. It was within these four walls that I became certain that there was nothing special about me. I was not as smart as I thought I was, as my mother taught me and made me believe I was. I wasn't even as tall as I thought I was. Medical school took away my own perception of myself and confirmed that I was indeed no god. I had spent my childhood lying to myself.

To learn within the walls of a medical school is to never be good enough. To always be made to feel like you are lacking the knowledge required to prove that you are worthy of the almighty title, "Dr." To learn within these walls is to live housed in fear, afraid of asking questions, challenging authority, changing the status quo. As we voraciously consume morsels of knowledge at lectures, ward rounds, emergency calls, we are unknowingly fed self-doubt. We are fed silence under the guise of obedience and respect—and we comply, to be found worthy in character. Like water poured into a black drum—for this is the shape I have learnt to take—I have become a question mark, my head bent always downward, my face to my chest, questioning my actions, my purpose, my existence. My journey with self-doubt is one that I hope ends when the light at the end of the tunnel bathes my face.

Within these walls too, forgetting is easy and ubiquitous. Remembering is difficult. You forget birthdays, names, indications for extractions and complications of mandibulectomies. Perchance the greatest thing that you forget—that I forgot—is that outside of these walls of the medical school, time still moves on. All my friends are working now, members of the hustle now, my young cousins are grown now and barely remember me. It seems I, on the other hand, am stuck, isolated in what seems like one spot: one level of learning teaches you to set teeth in the labs then morphs into learning to deliver them to the patient. You're still in the same hospital. Nothing has really changed.

But this is how I do (did) not break. I built a fortress in the lives of the characters of my favorite animes. I created alternate realities with my words, and escaped to places where I was still a god and my superpower was in my creating. I snuck into pages of novels and lines of poetry to get away from it all—the static, the noise that I was not good enough; the stress of course loads that seemed near impossible; the elusiveness of my memory. I heeded the words of Silken, "Everyone needs a place. It shouldn't be inside of someone else." So I left pieces of me with different people and created places in the things I love, and in the people who make my burden light. I am now your favorite adventure game: when time and life grab hold of someone I cherish and they leave, I rebuild with the places that remain. Nothing within these walls comes easy. Not breaking is my herculean labour.

This is me: the elusive memory, the crooked question mark, and the defiant piece. This is what I became within these walls. Even still, I am afraid that I will destroy the pieces of happiness that I have snatched from within these walls and hidden in those outside these walls by speaking it, by giving them names and breathing life to them on this page. There is a part of me, though—the part that remembers to be grateful for not being broken, for finding the people who eased my burden, for cold liquor on warm nights—that does feel indebted to these walls. It was within these walls that I gained the knowledge required to face the blinding light that awaits me at the end of the tunnel.

There are less than two months till I throw my exhausted body, and soul, over the finish line. No longer a boy, I have long since discarded the fantasies of capes and flight and am cursed to watch as time lords it over me. This is me: the elusive memory searching for a foothold in time, the defiant piece, the crooked question mark aiming to straighten out and challenge itself.

UCHECHUKWU O. | Nigeria

You Have Not Arrived

When they finally begin to notice,
and their eyes acknowledge the brilliance
your God has put between your ears,

When they finally start to twist their tongues
to the song that is your name,
and search for your voice when it is missing
from the conversation,

Embrace it.
Do not shrink back.

Speak with the eloquence of the women that have raised you.
Like your father, entrance them with the wisdom of your lips.
You are the sun. From you, light radiates.

But dear girl, lest you be tempted,
do not raise your shoulders higher than they ought to be.
The road ahead stretches farther than the eyes see,
and tall shoulders do weary a traveler.

Dear girl, lest you forget,
remind yourself,
you have not arrived.

TOLU K. | United States

You'll Become A Fine Doctor

During my internal medicine rotation as a third-year medical student, an attending physician asked me to take a history from an elderly man with hip pain and delirium. As I spoke with him, the patient drifted through various stages of consciousness, straying from my medical queries to describe instances in his life when he had been beaten and urinated on. A little confused, but under time pressure to complete the observed interview, I did my best to gently redirect him. That is, until he finally showed me a tattoo of coarse blue numbers on his forearm and said, "I was in Dachau for a while."

After his admission to the hospital, somebody informed the Holocaust survivor that the medical student on his care team was from Germany. Evidently it made an impression on him—despite his delirious state, he remembered this fact and from then on referred to me as "the German girl." I was afraid my presence would make his hospital stay unbearable, and would have understood if he had asked for me to be removed from the case. However, he was never anything but incredibly kind to me. I would visit him in the afternoon while waiting for admissions, and as his hip and mental status improved, he spoke less about his experiences inside the labor camps and instead told me the most incredible stories about his life after escaping to the US. Before the gentleman was discharged, he exhorted me to continue working hard and encouraged me, without having any objective evidence or indication of the fact: "You'll become a fine doctor one day."

This was an instance of a patient teaching me about compassion and humanism. He was willing to put aside not only history, but also his personal experiences during one of the most terrible atrocities of humankind, to get to know a random German medical student and encourage her. I learned three things. First, to never underestimate the value of "social rounds"—you will hear and learn the most fascinating things. Second, to always try to get to know the people around you even when your past experiences tempt you to put them in a "box." It will be easier to show the "opioid seeker," the "grumpy patient" or the "repeat ED admit" compassion if you know their story. Third, that encouragement is the most potent when it seems unwarranted. On the day you accidentally drop all your notes right before presenting, are blanking on your patients' names, and things seem like an irreversible mess, believe in yourself and remember, you'll become a fine doctor.

NATALIE R. | United States

Feb 3, 2016

Dr. Bailey being tied up in St. Mary's somewhere in Presidio, I had to run a mini-clinic and see four patients on my own, delving into a world of stasis ulcers, somatic symptom disorders, arteriovenous (AV) fistulas, and Hickman line evaluations. I cannot believe I was able to finish all encounters and come up with some assessments to relay to my attending.

Wear Una boots and elevate your legs. I care about
your bloodshot eyes, take good care, and come back to

re-evaluate. With positive thrills, let's get ultrasound run on your fistula to make sure flow is functional. I'll let her know, and let's schedule a follow up before your daptomycin ends its course.

Of course, I had help. Thank God for Claudia, Heather, and Keith. But this is about the very first time I've felt like I could pass as a future physician. The feeling is surreal. Ten years ago, I'm pretty sure I was studying for advanced placement Biology.

JIHAN R. | United States

Always Remember: A Letter to Medical Students, Interns, Residents, Fellows, and Junior Faculty

Dear Young Doctor,

As you go through your stages of training, know there will often be challenges and moments of self-doubt. And these moments hit harder at different stages for different people.

As a medical student who has been out of medicine or academia for a while, you might suffer from a severe case of "Imposter Syndrome." That feeling you have every time your colleagues mention something that you feel like you've never learned; the feeling of not even striving for honors, but just striving to be. Nobody talks about it but it's normal. Just accept you know relatively nothing, and that it's ok. Commit to an answer, even if it's wrong. Deep down, nobody truly expects you to know much of anything—there's a lot to learn.

As an intern, you're probably excited that now you get a pager, and you get to know almost everything going on with the patient. Enjoy that feeling while it lasts. Remember that feeling when it seems that everything is out of your control and nothing seems to be going right. For you too, just accept you know nothing, and that it's ok. Commit to an answer, even if it's wrong.

Nobody truly expects you to know anything, especially in your first few months. During those first few months, the senior resident is in charge anyway. A good one will have your back.

As the senior resident who just realized that something got missed, remember that that's ok too. It happens to all of us and you have faculty attendings, pharmacists, and everyone else on the team to look out for you. Keep pressing on.

As junior faculty, you're probably feeling a fair deal of trepidation that now the buck stops with you. Well, does it? You have an entire institution of people who've got your back. For you too, accept you don't know everything, and that it's ok. Commit to your decision, even if it feels shaky. Call a colleague, and get her opinion. Deep down, nobody truly expects you to know everything. There's still learning and growing to do.

No matter what stage you find yourself, it's ok to want to give up, ok to cry, ok to not want to go back. Cry it out. Talk it out. Pray it out. Remember who or what called you to it, and go back anyway.

SHERRY-ANN B. | United States

Remember

i have to find my confidence again
i gave it away, again
i forgot the pain
of the regret
that comes
with relinquishing my power

MOFIYIN O. | United States

Medicine: A Lifelong Journey

I've always wanted to be a physician. When I was little, I performed routine "checkups" on my teddy bears, and gave them "medications and vaccines" as necessary. As I grew older, I read as many medical books as I could, volunteered in medical clinics, and listened to the health portions of the news. I was amazed at the work physicians did. How was it, I thought, that doctors knew exactly what their sick patients needed to get better? I wanted to be that person; the person who helped physically fatigued people feel better or that lent a helping hand, open ears, and gentle heart when patients needed to vent and express their emotions. I wanted to use my knowledge and passion to better the world in any way possible. Medicine was where I belonged.

As you can imagine, the day I received my medical school acceptance email is one I will never forget. I remember my heart racing and my head getting light. I couldn't believe it! The little girl who pretended that her pens were vaccinations was finally going to become a doctor. A real doctor! As my medical education began, I quickly learned that medicine needed me to combine empathy and communication skills with expertise, clinical reasoning, and leadership. Medicine required me to work with other healthcare professionals and patients, and this meant that the interventions I performed would have to align with my patients' values, needs, and resources. I needed to be humble and to incorporate the best available evidence into all my decisions. The more I learned about medicine, the more I realized that there was much more to learn.

At times, this unending acquisition of knowledge made me love medicine even more. Other times however, it led to tremendous frustration that led me to question whether I had chosen correctly, whether I could truly be a good doctor someday. It was too much, too difficult: the studying, the memorization, the anatomy, the medications, the conditions, the breaking of bad news, the experiences of watching patients lose their battles.

But in those moments, my fears were quickly reversed when I would sit with a patient, listen to their story, and hear them tell me they felt relieved because they finally expressed their worries and emotions to someone. My uncertainty in my abilities were always replaced with confidence and hope. I may not be able to cure every patient I meet, but without a doubt, I will be a caring, intelligent, and empathetic doctor.

I'm discovering that good physicians are developed, not born. This lifelong journey of learning requires patience, but it is worth every minute it will take.

MARINA M. | Canada

FIVE

COPING

This is like being buried alive with a trowel.

Anonymous

Medical training is a marathon, with numerous trials dotting its course. Because human beings are highly adaptable, trainees find ways to survive, and even thrive, under the worst of conditions. In medicine, myriad stresses arise on both mind and body from dealing with human fragility daily or with the reality of onerous obligations. In this chapter, trainees reflect on the pressures of medical training and the mechanisms — positive or otherwise — that have helped them withstand these pressures.

A Dawn in Fog

Fog returned this morning
Made its way like an army up the river
and I rode with it downstream
as it lifted
slowly with the sun

KATHERINE F. | United States

The Trainee's Interface

Today I was a shoulder for many to cry on,
an undeserving confidante
relegated authority without concomitant merit,
a responsibility I'd rather be shared.

Today I was a double agent in the war between the doctor
    and the patient.
Privy to the judgmental attitudes of my seniors,
I remained sole witness to the ailing's darkest fears,
powerless as my advocacy fell on deaf ears.

This is the in-between, the dilemma,
the interface of the student:
not doctor enough to be consumed by orders that numb
    the soul,
but too layperson to be preserved from the emotional hazards
    of the occupation.

Yet I fear the day I will no longer "have the time" to be
    exposed to these tears;
The day Mrs. S's hand will no longer reach for mine,
her eyes bearing the pain of sleepless, spouseless nights;
or when I will be just a little too far away
to hear Mr. L croak, "Help me,"
as his lungs continue to fill with water;
or the day I do not realise that Miss M.
is one failing pain medication away from taking her life.
For it is in these moments of sacred vulnerability I find
    meaning.

Although it is challenging to brace this interface,
I am already mourning the transition to doctor,

the day my white coat will finally reach my knees,
as something tells me that both time and experience will
   continue to eat away
at the very thing that drew me to this profession.

SARAH H. | Canada

Sun Salutations

"No one lights a lamp and puts it in a place where it will be hidden, or under a bowl. Instead they put it on its stand, so that those who come in may see the light." (Luke 11:33, NIV)

"In Canada, the 'person' role was a late addition to the precursory work that informed CanMEDS, and was then excluded from the final set of CanMEDS role names." (Whitehead, Selleger, Kreeke, & Hodges, 2014)

I hear . . .

"It's all about work-life balance." He seesaws his white-coated arms, as if they are two pans of a scale rising and falling in op-position. More of life, less of work. More of work, less of life? Is that how it works? What then is life? And why do we work? When does life really start and when does it end?

Or, "I've got to put on my 'mom' hat for a minute!" she apolo-getically steps out of the patient room to take a phone call. ("It's the daycare asking for a change of briefs for my son, Max!") Was that a red ball-cap, a visor, or a scarf? Did she remove her "mom" hat after the call? What about the impression our hats leave—hat hair? Who are we at the end of the day when all our hats come off?

Or, "Do what you love and you won't work a day in your life." Then why do we live for the weekends, and make our living dur-ing the week? Is it because we take all the fun out of what we love, by working 100-hour weeks? Too much of anything will make you sick.

When I was on a rural placement in Northern Ontario, I became consumed by work. Though the January days were short, my days were long. From six a.m. to midnight, my thoughts revolved around medicine . . . chief complaints, physical exams, mnemonics, pathophysiology, differentials. The days began to blur together . . . one patient after another . . . one cup of coffee to the next . . . one article, and another . . . There was so much to learn, and I knew so little. If I was always toiling, I couldn't fall behind, right? I had to keep going.

One weary evening, as I was marching home from clinic, immersed in my relentless, restless mind, the brilliance of the setting sun caught my attention. Lifted from my reverie, I paused. I noticed:

The colours. Reds, oranges, and pinks, pirouetting across the horizon.

The cold wind. Tickling my cheeks.

The smell of smoke from burning wood stoves.

Galloping deer, crunching snow under their hooves.

A feeling of peace and acceptance filling me.

The experience of an invitation.

I felt inspired to create art. But first, I needed some supplies! Fortunately, the store in town was still open. Yes, pencil crayons would do just fine! I found a beautiful image of a meditating Buddha, with colours as rich as that setting sun. As I started to colour, I felt the warmth of effort radiate from my hand. The stress of the day drew away, the pressure of time released into the page, as I travelled into the meditating Buddha. My thoughts settled into the white noise of tracing, shading, scratching.

Shhh . . . ahhhh . . . I didn't know I was searching, but now I knew I had found what I was longing for.

The Buddha's golden face was the most challenging. There were so many shades needed to make it come alive. Black charcoal shadows at the jawbone's edge, gray, brown, mahogany, tan, orange, yellow-orange, peach, golden yellow, yellow . . . until the pure white light reflected off the cheekbone. Up close, my drawing looked like distinct colours side by side, but when I took a step back, the colours blended and a unified face emerged. So many colours, but still one face. Many individual qualities becoming one spiritual figure. As I adorned my statue in bright coloured garments, I felt brighter too. I could feel myself becoming whole.

Like a holy trinity, we are many things that are relationally one. We transcend our coats, our hats, our roles. Unashamed of our radiance, we shine.

DAPHNE D. | Canada

REFERENCE

Whitehead, C., Selleger, V., Kreeke, J., & Hodges, B. (2014). "The 'Missing Person' in Roles-Based Competency Models: A Historical, Cross-National, Contrastive Case Study." *Medical Education*, 48(8), 785–795.

Stress Dreams

After the first day, cold bodies fell on me all night long
Now my dreams are about your body and I stumble and fall
Soon they'll call me Doctor; maybe then my body will be in
    my dreams

CALEDONIA B. | United States

Taking A Drink From the Fire Hydrant

. . . It's like turning on a fire hydrant, and you are try-
ing to drink as much as possible out of it.

In my first week of medical school, I was constantly warned by my preceptors and friends about how heavy the medical curriculum was. There would be an overwhelming amount of information to be learned and what had worked at the undergraduate level might not work in medical school. Their advice? Accept that you won't be able to learn everything, and just try to find your flow in the system.

I didn't buy it. If I worked hard enough, I was sure I would be able to do as well as I had always done. I would simply have to be more efficient with my time. I cut time on social life and sleep to spend some extra time on studying. It worked perfectly well until I started to join different interest groups (and a recreational dodge ball team). My extracurricular activities demanded I cut down even more on sleep to keep up with studying. Not surprisingly, I ended up both physically and emotionally distressed from sleep deprivation. Unable to focus and spend my study time effectively due to a lack of sleep, I felt less fortunate and satisfied about the state of my life, and started to feel sorry for myself for not having the ability to perfectly balance everything.

When I felt like I couldn't take it anymore, I decided to close my lecture notes and call my mother. Although she was not an expert in medicine or mental health, she always actively listened to what I had to say over the phone. Whenever I shared my concerns with her, the fact that there was someone who I was able to completely share my inner frustrations with made me feel a lot better. At the end of the call, she asked, "If you have a patient who is completely devoting their life to work, what would you recommend?" Without a second thought, I told her that I would have an open discussion about the importance of having a balanced life: exercise, social life, family, and work. When she asked me why, I told her that focusing on one aspect of life would simply make the patient prone to a burnout. Then I had an epiphany; I was giving advice about lifestyle and behavior changes for patient wellness while ignoring them in my own life. I wasn't any different from physicians who advise their patients to quit smoking and then light up their cigarettes during a break.

Do we not recommend lifestyle and behavior changes targeting patient wellness while ignoring them in our own lives?

GLARA R. | Canada

Focus

Sometimes you get so focused
On the target and your goal
On ambitions and intentions
And fulfilling a set "role"

Sometimes you get so focused
On the science and "the fix"
You start to focus on diseases
Numbers, CBCs, and lists

Sometimes you get so focused
Really "in the zone"
You are having a conversation
But it's just with you alone

Sometimes you get so focused
You don't see the forest from the trees

The human from the ailment
The patient from the disease

Sometimes you get so focused
On what you are trying to do
That you forget about the journey
And learning from that too

Sometimes you get so focused
You forget about the human race—
Just like there's all kinds of people to treat
We need all sorts of doctors in this place

Sometimes you get so focused
Trying to fit into a mold
You forget about what makes you unique
And let your specialness unfold

Sometimes you get so focused
You forget that you are enough
That with compassion and understanding
You have all of the right stuff

Sometimes you need to remember
What it is you are trying to do
To focus on the journey
And bringing your best you

JENNIFER F. | United States

Fridays

Some Fridays start with a thank you
from a man in a blue gown, silver scalpel in hand.
Your retraction today, he says,
Stellar.

On these Fridays, acknowledgement from another,
similarly gowned, follows.
He actually looks you in the eye this morning.
Your talk, he says,
Well done.

Hours pass, then another gowned creature,
curved needle in hand, looks over to where your hands
have been busy with your own curved needle.
Your needlework, he says,
Beautiful.

These Fridays, make you stay.
These Fridays, you'll most definitely keep.

TOLU K. | United States

I Am Your Doctor

Knowledgeable, but never certain.
Schooled, but never finished.
Post-call, but never off.
Respected, but resented.
Well-paid, but hard price.
Expert, but unemployed.
Confident, but questioning.
Committed, but cannot say no.

Compassionate, but concealed.
Good, but never good enough.

I am a doctor, yet

I am a worker, longing for rest.
I am an explorer, longing to find.
I am a chef, longing to please.
I am a poet, longing to muse.

I am a doctor, yet

I am a daughter, longing for guidance.
I am a woman, longing to mother.
I am a wife, longing to settle.
I am a sibling, longing to play.

I am a doctor, yet

I am a river, longing to run.
I am a moon, longing to shine.
I am a breeze, longing to sing.
I am a ship, longing to sail.

I am
Lost and yearning and
      Artistic and growing and
      Heard and known and
      Serious and funny and
Bright and colorful and strong and
      Tired and awake and dreaming and
      Burning and quiet and confident and
          Precise and perceptive and
      Steady and wild and
Well-paid and generous and

Young and grey and
　　Wise and free and

and I am your doctor.

MOIRA H. | Canada

Balance

A rare occurrence, but today, I needed a moment. I excused myself, walked into the bathroom, shut the door behind me and let my tears flow. I cried for a few minutes, then dried my eyes. I stopped at the kitchen on labor and delivery, got a cold drink, and headed back to work.

I am thirty-six weeks pregnant, an Obstetrician and Gynecology (OB/GYN) resident, working eighty hours a week, and the chief resident for the Labor and Delivery rotation this month. I feel exhausted. The notion that we as women can do it all is highly advertised, but I've come to realize that in the "doing" there will be laughter, tears, aches and pains—the study of medicine can completely consume one's life. But giving your life to the mastery and betterment of the human body does seem like a worthy cause. In the end, it will all be worth it.

Yes, I choose to be a physician, specifically an OB/GYN, but I also choose to be a wife and a mother. The latter two being the most important things I will ever do in life. Thus, my task has become mastering the balance. I do love my job, but I'm learning to see it as one compartment. The same type of focus, development, and attention given at work is also deserved in one's personal life. Well-rounded lives make us better people and better physicians.

OLUBUNMI A. | United States

... If Just For A Little While

i knew a man who died yesterday.

it'd almost been a year since i'd seen him last. it was a quick
visit.
i went with his oldest son who said
he had always asked about me.

i met him when i was seventeen,
introduced to him by S.

i remember that he made me laugh and bubble at his
compliments.
but now, i grieve for the pain embracing his loved ones.

i didn't see the sun today. i had a long shift
working, as an intern,

at a children's hospital,
where i thought about death,
but kept it professional.

tammi c. | United States

In A Bubble of Happiness

What makes you who you are? Is it the ability to express yourself
in eloquent words in the language of your choosing? Is it the
ability to decide what your day will be like, or what meal you will
have next? Is it being able to go to school, get an education, and
decide what sort of job you would like to have one day? Or is it
being able to decide, upon the sensation of a full bladder, when
to allow your urethral sphincters relax and allow urine pass?

Today was my fourth visit to a daycare centre for mentally disabled children. The centre serves twenty kids, most of whom suffer from cerebral palsy, foetal alcohol syndrome, or autism. When my group was first assigned to this place as part of our community health project, I knew that this would be challenging for me: I would not cope well around sick or disabled children. But I figured that while I would struggle, I would eventually do well. How wrong I was.

There was nothing special about today. The same kids I had met on previous visits were there, and neither the caregivers nor my group members had changed. I always tried to push myself to be as playful with the children as I could possibly be, but today, I struggled a great deal. A child to my left, strapped in her wheelchair was crying her eyes out, clearly agitated. With the little movement her body allowed, she tried to worm her way out of the chair. I wanted to help, but as she could not communicate what was wrong or what she needed, I was helpless. Behind me, another girl, who could only roll on the floor and was no older than three, hit her head against a wall. She didn't cry or fuss. She simply rolled over to another place. Nearby, an eleven-year-old boy with a staggering gait and minimal arm movements sat in my colleague's lap. The boy did nothing out of character, but unable to vocalise words, continued to scream as he had done since the first time we met him. On a small plastic chair next to mine, another boy, severely autistic, sang beautifully with another of my colleagues. As I sat there taking everything in, my eyes caught the three-year-old girl with Spina Bifida, and paralysis below the knee, sitting close by. I thought about how her chances to lead a successful life would be much better in a place that was better suited for her, a place where she could learn and read books and imagine a better future for herself.

I had never really been exposed to children with disabilities before, and the fact that so much stigma exists around people living with disabilities wasn't much help either. I firmly believe that people can change the course of their lives, but as I looked at these children, I was disheartened; it seemed very little could be done to change their fates. They should be given as much support as possible to ensure they lived lives not predetermined by their limitations. But unfortunately, in a country like South Africa, where money is not always available, this isn't always possible. I wondered if these children had ever dreamt of a different life, but then again, closed off from the world, how would they know to dream of any life different from theirs? I tried to fake a smile, but instead a tear fell onto my lap. I knew I could not stay there. I would not be the one to dampen the bubble of happiness that these children lived in.

MBULELO K. | South Africa

Retained Guilt

New phase, new place, same journey,
and like in the past, those who look the most like me,
are not with me.

Reflections are in the cleaners and wipers,
Thirty-two gallons and grey, hazardous and red, in tow.
Give the nod, add a faint smile.
Must acknowledge my reflections.

Don't want to feel the need
to overcompensate,
to atone,
for a wrong that is not mine.
Free me
to stand tall, shoulder-to-shoulder
with those who look the most like me.

MOFIYIN O. | United States

The Stuff of Nightmares

Sometimes, I am still at work while I sleep.

One night, instead of visions of sugar plums, I dreamed of endless loops of bowel and globs of sticky blue mucin; then, of long bones, still warm, in my two hands.

Another night, I tried to keep an extremely premature fetus safe by tucking it away in my sweatshirt pocket. Then, I went for a bike ride, forgetting the guest I was housing. It was only at the end of the ride, when I reached into my pocket, that I discovered it had died. A delicate leg broke off. I returned it to its mother, profusely apologizing.

On yet another night, I found myself in the autopsy suite when a body was wheeled in from the operating room, covered in a white sheet. Left for dead. A faceless voice warned me: *We're leaving this here, DON'T bring it back.* Then there was movement from beneath the sheet. *Still alive!* Fear struck my heart but I stamped it out as I approached the gurney. The patient was a young woman. "I don't feel so good," she said with a grimace. As I found the courage to sit by her side, I realized I was more afraid of someone who was dying than someone who was dead.

DIANE B. | United States

Conflicted

"Are you still enjoying medicine?"

The doctor asked at the end of the lecture. Yeses erupted around me. I wanted to join in but words choked in my throat. I wanted to affirm my boundless love for medicine, but I couldn't. Just two days prior, a four-month-old baby was brought into the trauma unit from a house that had burnt down. No one else was injured. The baby sustained full-thickness burns on fifty-five percent of its body with significant inhalation burns. He died the next morning in ICU. Another patient, a fifty-one-year-old man, who I met the other day and who reminded me of my own father, languished away as stomach cancer ravished his body. Earlier that day, I had to tell a forty-two-year-old diabetic woman, in need of an amputation for over a month, that again, like yesterday, the theatre could not accommodate her.

I actually enjoy the long hours I spend at the hospital. I am incredibly grateful that I get to see patients, interact with them and integrate lecture-room knowledge to clinical practice. I am living my childhood dream and get to inspire other young black kids to be fearless in the pursuit of their dreams. But how do you not absorb your patients' situations into yours? How do you hold your head high, when you come bearing news that shatters hope? How do you continue to pour yourself out to others, even when it means sacrificing time with your own family and friends, the people you owe so much to?

I don't think I could ever hate medicine, but the rhetoric that one must struggle for what one loves is proving true.

MBULELO K. | South Africa

SIX

MISTAKES AND NADIRS

Sometimes you want to land the broken plane.
Sometimes you want to ride it to its inevitable crash.
Anonymous

Stakes are high when human lives are concerned. Mistakes in medicine can range from awkward to incredibly costly. The stresses of medical training can also plunge trainees into the depths. In this chapter, trainees reflect on mistakes they've witnessed as well as low points in their training.

Untitled

Kicking yourself
because you made a mistake.
Knowing
they make mistakes too.
Yet
wondering

whether your mistake will be reduced to eye rolls and
   "... affirmative action,"
and theirs,
compassionate gazes and "... humanness."

ANONYMOUS | United States

Finding Humanity

Days in the surgical intensive care unit (SICU) as a medical student were often dull and repetitive, amounting to hours of sporadically educational rounds with droning dialogue about medication dosing, rate-control for arrhythmias, and discharge planning. After rounds, I would often stare at the antiquated computer monitor for hours and pray that my supervising residents would send me home. Medical or surgical emergencies, while occurring more frequently in an ICU, are still not as ubiquitous as television would make them appear. What "action" did transpire often occurred in the late evening or early morning when medical students were at home respecting duty-hour regulations.

It was a standard July day in the SICU as a fourth-year sub-intern: sign-out from the night team and pre-rounds on our patients followed by formal rounds from eight a.m. until my soul was taken to Valhalla or lunch, whichever came first. Admissions to the SICU were of two varieties: planned postoperative admissions for patients requiring precautionary monitoring and transfers from the general floor for patients whose health had become tenuous. However, today was different. An unanticipated patient appeared on the electronic medical record's track board and a surprise admission could only mean one thing—perioperative complications. But this admission was peculiar. The gentleman in question was a previously healthy man with no comorbidities and was scheduled to undergo a laparoscopic right nephrectomy for an insidiously enlarging renal cell carcinoma (RCC). The operation should have been quick and uncomplicated; if all had gone as planned, he would have been discharged home within twenty-four hours. But obviously, this operation did not go as anticipated. Being far-removed from the operating room on the upper floors of the towering hospital, I gathered information second- and third-hand as quickly as I could. I learned that the surgical team had encountered intraoperative hemorrhage necessitating massive blood product transfusion. I also learned that the vascular surgery team was consulted, came to the operating suite and attempted to repair the damaged vessel and temper the bleeding, but the patient's condition remained critical.

When I first saw the patient, he was intubated, sedated, pale, and seemingly lifeless. His pulse was barely palpable, and his blood pressure was rapidly plummeting. Despite the multiple transfusions and operative intervention, he was coagulopathic and still hemorrhaging. A "blood alert" was called and the other medical students and I took shifts running through the hospital, down old hallways, and through service corridors to manually deliver coolers of blood products to the SICU. His abdomen rapidly became grotesquely engorged as each transfused unit seeped through his broken vasculature into his stomach. After what seemed like an eternity of this hurried and feverish activity, we noticed the patient's wife on the periphery: she stood behind the nurses' station, a look of shocked disbelief on her face. The intensive care physician and the vascular surgeon paused to talk with her.

The vascular surgeon stood with the wife and calmly stated the facts: her husband had suffered an intraoperative injury and, despite our attempts to remedy his blood loss, he was exsanguinating faster than we could transfuse him. In plain words, he noted, "We can attempt to open his stomach and repair the injury, or we can let him pass in peace: either way, he will likely not leave the hospital." This seemed to me, a kind way of noting that medical care was likely not going to save her husband; but it was also a way of deferring to her agency, as his wife and companion, regarding his last moments. Still in disbelief, she replied, "I understand what you're saying, but I think you should at least try to fix the problem. I just don't understand how this happened — he was gardening just yesterday."

I could only imagine the horror she was experiencing. Was she recalling images of an otherwise healthy husband, father, and grandfather? Or recalling the pre-surgical outpatient visit where the words, "routine," "quick," and "painless," were uttered along with the disclaimer that he'd be "back to himself in no time." Was she remembering the waiting room where all families experience some degree of fear while their loved one undergoes an operation? She may have been revisiting the call from the circulating nurse that informed her of the complication. And through it all, there was the haunting image of her bloated, battered, and fileted husband on the table, surrounded by countless individuals working to curb the tide of blood loss. And she was helpless.

Within minutes, sterile equipment, drapes, and gowns appeared and the room was converted into an operating suite. As the closest to the door, I donned sterile attire and wedged myself behind the vascular surgeon. After a quick midline laparotomy, an incalculable volume of blood poured down the bed, onto the floor, and into my shoes. The patient's most central pulses became faint, then disappeared entirely, and the closest person to the bedside became responsible for constant chest compressions as the vascular surgeon once again attempted to repair the injury. After thirty minutes, he was declared dead.

I pulled off my gown and gloves and began to help clean the room so the patient's wife would not have this apocalyptically bloody scene as the last image of her husband. Many of the other medical students, nurses, and residents choked back tears; others let them flood freely. Once the room was cleaned, we brought the wife in. She kissed her husband on the forehead, and, after conferring with the physicians one last time, left the hospital.

What had just happened? A perfectly healthy man had just lost his life. A husband, a father, and someone who could have been a businessman, a scientist, or a poet now lay dead in the hospital morgue. I was disturbed that I knew almost nothing about this man and equally disconcerting was the leviathan of responsibility I felt for his outcome. I wanted to be a surgeon, and I had just witnessed the devastation caused by a simple surgical error. Moreover, I realized that such an experience would likely occur during my surgical training, requiring me to look someone in the eye and say, "I made a mistake. I'm so sorry." But didn't I already know this? Wasn't it common knowledge? That's why our patients sign consent forms, right? As the French surgeon René Leriche wrote, "Every surgeon carries about him a little cemetery, in which from time to time he goes to pray, a cemetery of bitterness and regret, of which he seeks the reason for certain of his failures."

I grappled with the syncretic juxtaposition of the "glorious" field of surgery and the dark reality of how some patients would suffer, struggle, and die in our care. But, I also reflected on how selflessly and tirelessly the care team fought in the face of insurmountable odds. It would be an honor, I thought, to be the last resort, the person willing to try anything if it meant saving one additional life. Yes, I would still train to be a surgeon, but this incident would be the first gravestone in a cemetery that reminded me of the humanity of my patients — and myself.

This experience has taught me important lessons about life and how to be a better physician. I know there will be moments when I'm scared, unsure, or simply ignorant. I know there will be patients and families whose outcomes I cannot guarantee. But, aware of the devastating consequences of mistakes, I'm comfortable setting pride aside and asking for help. It can be easy to view each patient as a "case" bantered about with jargon that is limited to pathophysiology and operative maneuvers. Obviously, some degree of detachment is necessary when we care for the suffering, but humanity cannot be cast aside. I trust I'll never forget that each patient is a person with a story, a unique life, and a circle of family and friends who love, cherish, and depend on them. With pride and humility, I will take responsibility for being a patient's physician and appreciate the trust patients have in me.

Balancing the ability to treat and sometimes cure disease with the risk of hastening death is a fundamental tenet of physician-hood. I can't begin to articulate or even postulate how we should reconcile this age-old conflict of our profession, but I can advocate for a moment of reflection each day to consider the humanity of our patients, our colleagues, our subordinates, and all those working to heal others through medicine. Take a moment to remember that everyone has a story we may not be considering before it's too late, as I did. Whether its understanding their history, their heritage, or recognizing their significant other as they stand on the periphery in disbelief, viewing people as human beings, just like ourselves, is a challenge to take a step forward. And although this simple act won't immediately solve any world crises, it may make today a better day than yesterday.

JOSHUA J. | United States

REFERENCE

Leriche R. *La philosophie de la chirurgie.* Paris: Flammarion, 1951

Foamy

On one of my visits to my preceptor's office, I interviewed the parents of a pediatric patient. When I had the information I needed about their child's symptoms, I summarized the pertinent findings I had heard back to them to make sure I hadn't missed anything. I relayed that the mother had mentioned that the child's mouth was foamy, but the father immediately corrected me saying that this was never mentioned. I was taken aback. I was pretty certain she had mentioned foamy, and not just once, but twice, in fact. Thoughts sloshed around my mind. *Wait, did I just mishear her? No, no, I am pretty sure she said foamy. Maybe I am sleep deprived, I thought she said the child was foamy while pointing to the kid's mouth.* To stop the market in my head, I quickly apologized, adding that I must have misheard them. This was after all why the summary at the end of the interview was so important. I carried on with the rest of my summary, clarifying questions that came up.

"Oh, I think she was saying fome! As in he/she is fome. Hungry."

I looked at them, confused. The father continued on to explain that "fome" meant "hungry" in Portuguese and that the child's mother was trying to convey that he seemed to be hungry/fome. It all finally made sense.

This encounter reinforced the importance of summarizing details back to patients at the end of interviews. It also reminded me that so much of medicine and good patient care require clear communication between physicians and patients.

NAYAN A. | United States

What Medical School Has Taught Me

For as long as I can remember, I have wanted to be a medical doctor. Working feverishly towards this goal, I did well at school, pursued research, volunteered wherever I could. So understandably, when I found myself on my dream school's waitlist, I was disappointed. But determined still, I chose to enroll at a school that had been at the bottom of my safety school list, in a country I honestly didn't know existed prior to applying. This was a low point, but I had no idea how much lower things were about to get in medical school.

Starting out, my strategy was to just get my work done. There would be no socializing because I just needed to put my head down and get through as quickly as possible. And for a while, this worked: I did well in school. But while I was used to being the outstanding student, I soon realised that I was surrounded by equally outstanding students and I quickly fell into the vortex of comparison. As I wallowed, my disappointment in myself—that I hadn't made it to my dream school, that I was now in fact in a Caribbean school, that I was in fact not the most brilliant in the room—grew.

It was at this low point that I somehow drew closer to God. And as I prayed and journaled, and prayed and journaled, I found myself asking less whether I would ever be good enough. Journaling reminded me of the passion that first drove me to medicine and gradually, I no longer wanted to just survive—I wanted to thrive. I started to see my current situation as an opportunity to learn about navigating life's disappointments.

So far, medical school has taught me:

- To compare yourself to others is to suffocate yourself and stunt your growth.
- Where people are fickle, God is as sure as the dawn.
- Sticky notes and constant self-encouragement can be life-giving.

- Even beyond exams and tests, plan for the doctor you want to become.
- Yes, you will sleep when you're dead, but to really live, you must rest.
- What has happened has happened. Make the most of now.

ENE M. | Grenada

Broken

On a lovely December evening, I returned to my apartment to find my roommate weeping. For the three years I have known her, I have respected her for her strength — nothing could scare or intimidate her. When no one else would, whether for shyness or apathy, she would be the person to stop a lecture to raise an important question or ask the professor to clarify a point. Her fearlessness endeared her to our classmates. So, when on that day, I was greeted by loud sobs coming from her room, I knew something significant had happened: medicine had finally broken her. It was really the only thing that could. Eventually, all of us break down.

I wondered how a profession sworn to bring healing could be so adept at destroying the wills of the ones that had answered its call. I knew what my friend was going through because I had experienced it multiple times. Medicine tells you that your best is never good enough, that perfection is required of you. The barrage of evaluations and criticisms is unending, as you are constantly asked to do better, read more, practice more, take care of more patients, speak up more. Medicine is a treadmill that exhausts you, pinning you down till getting off becomes even harder than getting on.

As my friend's sobs continued, I was at a loss for what to do. I knew words were helpless. This is what medicine does. This is medicine. So, rather than speak, I knocked on her door, and sat with her, all the while praying she would recover from this and all the while doubting she ever would. None of us do.

PEACE E. | United States

SEVEN

PHYSICIAN, HEAL THYSELF

The body takes what it needs.

Anonymous

Medical professionals are tasked with alleviating suffering in others. Our gaze is constantly outwards. But what happens when the healer is broken? How do you keep looking outwards, when inside is riddled with grief from the loss of a loved one, disappointment, or with actual disease? In this chapter, medical trainees reflect on personal struggles with physical and mental health. Some discuss the role medical culture has played in uncovering their struggles, others tell how these struggles now fit into the trainees' own medical journeys and enhance patient interactions.

Fighting Flight

Fighting flight:
Fight flying
Moving slow
Staying away
Staying low

Staying in
Staying safe and warm and close
Then
Same and same and same
Then
Stifled and stuffy and closed

Going out

Getting up
Breaking off
Taking off
Fight fleeing:
Fighting flight

GLORIA O. | United Kingdom

Snow Day

It's mid-afternoon on a Tuesday. I'm wearing pajamas and sitting on my couch with my tuxedo cat buried deep in my lap—
not a typical day for an internal medicine intern. It's March in
Boston, and outside my window there is heavy snow falling,
high winds howling, and large trucks plowing. On this bliz-
zard day, I somehow manage to be scheduled to the only shift
in residency that is non-essential. With only three patients of
moderate acuity at the Veteran's Association (VA) intensive care
unit, my long call team has offered me the day off.

You might guess that I'm feeling overjoyed at this opportunity
to sleep in, watch television, and stuff myself with leftover birthday cake. I am indeed contemplating these activities, but elation
does not exactly describe my current emotion. I feel clogged with
panic.

My co-residents are completing their afternoon tasks on patients I cared for yesterday, including an eighty-nine-year-old
who will likely pass away during this storm. My fiancé is in the
hospital serving an oncology service and won't be home until
later in the evening—if he can even make it through the snow.
Our second-year residency schedule was just released, placing
my first rotation as a supervising resident in the scariest place
in the hospital—the cardiac intensive care unit. I am already
feeling unprepared for that dreaded moment and am lamenting
that today will be a day without learning and practice. I just don't
feel like I deserve this day off.

This feeling is not unfamiliar to me. Sometimes I call it guilt,
sometimes anxiety. It has been around me and inside me for
some time. As a thirteen-year-old, for an English assignment
in which I was asked to describe my superstitions, I described
it as "an evil cloud, living right below my ribs sending vibes out
everywhere." It is the feeling that something is just not quite
right. In clinical terms, it is my depression. And medical school
was the first time I named it as such.

My depression is episodic—sometimes fleeting, and sometimes hanging on for days or weeks. While it has been smol-
dering within me since childhood, medical training gave it the
ground to blossom. When I entered medical school, I hopped
onto that conveyer belt that doesn't stop moving, doesn't toler-
ate weakness or hesitancy, and doesn't allow space for grieving
or loss. And with that momentum, I lost the ability to care for
myself in the ways that I needed.

I hit my low when I took a year off for research and I was no
longer frantically filling each moment of my day with a check
box. It surfaced when I had a chance to sit down and read fic-
tion, a moment to learn a new recipe, and the time to think up
a hobby. It was the first time in years that I was forced to face
myself—rather than focusing on the tasks ahead of me in the
next hour, and the steps ahead of me in the next years.

I spent many hours crying and finding fault with myself. At my worst moments, I hit my temples with the palms of hands and fantasized about the sharp blade of the kitchen knife. I was a bad daughter, a bad partner—and someday I would be a bad mother. While I had once known I would be a good doctor, I now questioned this notion immensely. I had entered a career path where good was never good enough. And I was surrounded by people too tired to care for themselves, much less give me the immense reassurance I suddenly needed from everyone around me that I was going to be ok.

This was my secret life. Outside my home and my relationship, I put on a show. I presented myself as competent and energetic, and boasted a sarcastic but compassionate sense of humor. I ran the student wellness group, and spoke publicly about the risky intersections of mental health and medical school. My goal was for no one to imagine that I was in a dark place myself. And thus, I perpetuated the stigma that everyone entering medicine confronts on those days in which they just can't muster being perfect.

I sought help. I leaned on a therapist for weekly consultation. I started a medication that helped me weather the ups and downs. I leaned on a small group of friends from whom I kept nothing. And I relied on my partner, whose patience and love were tested every day. Day-by-day, the darker moments got shorter. I anticipated the plummets and learned to call them out before they consumed me. And while I believe I have recovered from my worst symptoms, I imagine my depression will always lurk within me. When my world quiets down, it finds a path to resurface—like a potential space whose physiology is as predictable as a beating heart.

These days in residency, each moment is filled with one, two, or three tasks at a time. I write my notes while on hold. While my patient shares extraneous details, I check his labs at his bedside. While I put in orders, I eat my lunch and respond to a nurse's concern behind me without even turning my head. Yet when there are seconds to spare, I am often filled with the dread that I am missing something, that I've made a mistake that will harm my patients, or that I am somehow letting down my peers around me. Because even when the task in front of me is literally impossible, I am expected to complete it. To ask for help is demoralizing. To admit I need a moment of rest or recuperation, unthinkable.

I will never know if my fear of a snow day would have emerged if I had not become a doctor. However, I do know that medicine imbeds self-doubt into even the most confident, pessimism into the most positive, and worry into the care-free. I know that medical training has taken far too many young lives, whose exhaustion and sense of inadequacy grew too great to bear. And I know that despite my daily decision to trudge on, I too am not immune to contemplating the tempting relief of escaping it all.

KATHERINE B. | United States

Needles and Insulin

Every day for the past two years, I have medically managed one long-term patient with a chronic life-threatening condition. I collect daily bloodwork, administer hourly medications, adjust dosages, triage symptoms, and coordinate care among insurance companies, medical device suppliers, and doctors' offices. I was there when he was unexpectedly diagnosed in the hospital, when he administered his first of thousands of injections, and when he realized that he had been taking his healthy years for granted. I also observed as he learned everything he could about his disease, taught others what he discovered, and used his situation as a way to better understand what it's like to be sick.

While I could not have imagined it at the time, being diagnosed with Type 1 diabetes in my first year of medical school was actually a gift to my education. I experienced the uncertainty and sadness that comes with a new diagnosis, the sensation of losing control of normal bodily functions, and the helpless feeling of lacking access to care when it's needed the most. On the other hand, I also celebrated my progress, established a strong support network, and cultivated resilience that will sustain me through future challenges. In a system where it is expected that the healthy care for the sick, I wonder how patient care can be improved when doctor is also patient.

As I get to know my patients, I now view their journey from a new perspective. I can empathize with the disappointment of receiving a discouraging lab value despite working diligently for improvement. I understand just how vulnerable and uncertain it feels when the need for a diagnosis is met with a dry list of possible differentials and more questions. I now appreciate how illness reaches beyond the patient and can also affect his or her family and friends. Most importantly, I know that the person in front of me is so much more than just a list of problems; what we see in the hospital or clinic is only a sliver of what patients experience every day.

JOHN M. | United States

Through the Dark

What you read in books or see in movies is true: medical school is tough. It stretches you mentally, physically, socially—and nobody leaves unscathed.

In my fifth year, I discovered my first lymph node. My classmates and I had been preparing for an exam and to reinforce my general examination skills. I decided to practice on myself, reaching to my neck to palpate the lymph nodes there. I pressed my hand into the angle between my jaw and neck, and felt a single lymph node. I thought nothing of it. Submandibular lymph nodes could become prominent from mild illness local to the area. But the lymph node never resolved, and with time, two more appeared with it. At the time, I had lost some weight and was battling constant fatigue, but I was stressed about exams and was sleeping very little, so those symptoms made sense. I tried to shake off thoughts that something might truly be wrong with me.

Exams came and went, but the nodes were steadfast and I wasn't feeling any better. A general blood workup showed mildly low haemoglobin levels but everything else was normal. Mild anemia could explain my constant tiredness and the breathlessness I had recently started to feel. I rested easy for a while, but as time went on, classmates started to comment on how skinny I had gotten and former lecturers would cast surprised glances in my direction in the corridors. As I noticed I wasn't regaining any of my lost weight, the worry that something was seriously wrong with me grew. Trying to balance school at the same time made me even more of an emotional mess.

A few months passed, and then recurrent fevers started. This time, I chalked it up to stress, or maybe malaria. But my symptoms worsened, and despite iron supplements, my haemoglobin levels continued to decline. And then, surprisingly, after my final medical school exams, the fevers stopped and I seemed to have a little more energy. I tried to convince myself that the worst was over. But in retrospect, I was by no means out of the woods. If anything, that brief period was the quiet before the storm.

The storm came at the end of my internship year. It started with a seemingly routine cold, which later progressed to a bad cough and a long period of illness. Once more, I was back in labs for more blood work and, this time around, X-rays and scans. The results of these tests were still unrevealing but, totally weakened by this point, I took six weeks off work. That had to be the most trying time of my life so far: lying in my hospital bed, my body trembling from fevers, there were many times I thought I wouldn't make it.

Much later, it was discovered that the problem all along was that my immune system was at war with my body. I had never really appreciated the importance of good health up until then. The fact is, as doctors, although we are surrounded by sickness, we don't always fully understand our patients' weakness and vulnerability till we find ourselves in similar situations. In the throes of illness, I initially thought that if I ever got better, I would walk away from medicine and find a different career path. But I now realise that my experience will likely make me a better doctor. I often wonder if the stresses of medical school triggered my illness, whether my symptoms would have surfaced if I had chosen a different profession. If I was in medicine, perhaps I would have taken better care of myself, had more time *for* myself. But through this process I have rediscovered the joys of living and learned from the challenges of building from scratch. I still have doubts about whether medicine is the right path but for now, I choose to channel the lessons I have learned to helping my patients heal and work through disease.

ANONYMOUS | Nigeria

Where Do Broken Hearts Go?

At the beginning of medical school, every single professor made one thing very clear: we were to leave our emotional baggage behind. If a thought or relationship did not make us perform at our best every single day, we could not afford to waste time on it in medical school. I heard them loud and clear. I saw many classmates fall behind and spiral into bad places because they didn't let go of their baggage. I didn't want to be *that* person. There was just too much on the line and my parents had invested a ridiculous amount of time, effort, and money in my education. *I* had invested everything. But while I didn't want to be *that* person, or think I was *that* person, the truth was I had just gotten out of a relationship, one that had spanned the entirety of college. Truth is, people don't just get over things they once cared deeply about.

Medical school doesn't give you a lot of time to deal with heartbreak. Regardless of the state of your heart, it continues, relentless, quizzing you on every detail of the body, then of potential mishaps, then of remedies. It doesn't ask about the guy you fell in love with in college and can't get over. Or how you feel about it. But the rest of life does. I'd find myself reminded of him when a song I thought he might like came up on my playlist as I studied. When I learned about new diseases or intriguing tidbits, I'd think about sharing my new knowledge with him. He was in medical school after all, and might have liked to know that red-orange urine could be from Rifampin, and not necessarily hematuria. In those moments, I'd think of the emptiness inside, the closure I never got, and of Kate Winslet's lines from *The Holiday*:

> "I understand feeling as small and as insignificant as humanly possible. And how it can actually ache in places you didn't know you had inside you. And it doesn't matter how many new haircuts you get, or gyms you join, or how many glasses of Chardonnay you drink with your girlfriends . . . you still go to bed every night going over every detail and wonder what you did wrong or how you could have misunderstood. And how in the hell for that brief moment you could think that you were that happy. And sometimes you can even convince yourself that he'll see the light and show up at your door . . ."

But medical school keeps asking of you. Despite your feelings, it asks you to embrace the right amount of confidence and poise, asks you to radiate humility and brilliance. So when, in one day, your thoughts jump from "oh-my-god-i'm-totally-at-my-best-nothing-can-ever-bring-me-down!" to "i'm-so-devastated-and-will-never-come-out-of-this," you train yourself to ignore these thoughts and think logically, because that is what is required of you in medicine. You see people go through heartbreak every day—from the loss of a loved one, the loss of an arm in war, the inevitable fading of a child with metastatic cancer. But you also see many emerge on the other side—no one ever dies from heartbreak.

I no longer find myself thinking of all the things we did wrong, or all the things that made me want to hate him so badly after the way things ended. I no longer find myself recalling all the things he said and did that broke my heart. I no longer find myself asking, "What if I did this . . ." or "If only I said that . . ." Medical school puts things in perspective, teaches you about yourself, shows you how to move on.

"And after all that, however long all that may be, you'll go somewhere new. And you'll meet people who make you feel worthwhile again. And little pieces of your soul will finally come back. And all that fuzzy stuff, those years of your life that you wasted, that will eventually begin to fade . . ."

RIDDHI D. | United States

Depth

When I can no longer see the sun, like a swelling tide you
    come crashing over walls.
Yet the storm is no less when you're gone,
your destruction leaving behind shards and weakened pieces of
    my guard.
To you, goodbye I shall not say, for I know you will return
    when I least expect.
Your hold covers me whole. I shudder as I sense your grasp
    tighten;
how like vines to trees, you suffocate the soul.
You are all encompassing and rule my thoughts. Each day I
    awaken more and more numb.

While I wait this particular phase out, Love and its power
    have left me for now.
Deeper and darker the days get and further into the depths I
    sink,
gasping for air
wishing, praying,
for this misery to end.

And then suddenly you are gone.
The sun is up, a new day has come. My breath has returned as
    if nothing was done.
Leap, I must at the chance to be one determined to bloom.
Still, deep inside I know what's true,
that one day to the fray I will be returned.

SAHIL B. | United States

Upwards and Onwards

"Everyone has a coping mechanism." A third-year law student
said that to me my first week in Bloemfontein. What he didn't
tell me though was that for some of us, said coping mechanism
would be a chemical concoction.

When I first came to university, I wasn't sure whether I
wanted to be a doctor. Were four or five years of fire worth it?
Many of my classmates were drawn to medicine for altruistic
reasons, but for me, money was the lure. And it was a powerful
lure: I decided quickly that four or five years of fire were indeed
worth it. Besides, I was black, with black parents. Which black
parent didn't want a doctor for a kid? Heck, my grandmother
was even already telling her coworkers that I was a doctor.

I wasn't worried about medicine initially. I had made it after
all. What would follow would simply be formalities. But was I

wrong! I have never had my ass handed to me as bad as it has been in medicine. There have been weeks I have forgotten to eat, others when I have studied with tonsils bigger than lemons and still more when I haven't been able to get any work done at all. My days have been largely unpredictable, but a few things have been constants: mental breakdowns, explanations of said breakdowns to my black parents, a perennial sense of sticking out like a sore thumb, and perpetual financial insolvency.

My first breakdown was last June, just before my first set of exams in university. I had had what had been the most difficult semester of my life and I couldn't shake the feeling that I was going to fail. To make matters worse, I fell ill five days before my most difficult exam: Psychology. It was a horrible week, but somehow, I pulled through, but that week started a long term relationship with the faculty shrink—I am currently on SSRIS and Ritalin.

Telling my parents was difficult. I could hear my mum's silence from 400 km away when I finally called her. I couldn't see her, but I knew what the look on her face would say: confusion, disappointment, disbelief. How could her first-born, her golden boy, the center of her world be depressed? Depression is something the black community equates to being a "white people problem." It doesn't matter whether you are from the fourth world or a doctorate holder like my mum, this just never happens to black people. Never.

I, for one, still struggle with this diagnosis. How do you explain depression to yourself and how do you explain it to someone else when you yourself aren't really sure about the details? Will it end? Was it caused by something in my upbringing?

Several months in, answers still elude me. So I have found ways to cope: girls, Ceylon tea, other things for which I could be arrested. This is the only way I move forward because the destination has to be reached, at any cost and by any means. In medicine, you find what drives you and use it, whether it is the alleviation of suffering, self-fulfillment, or the Mercedes-Benz that is waiting. It is impossible to leave medical school the same way you entered. Something will get you. But you have to keep moving. In medicine, it is always upwards and onwards, onwards and upwards.

TAKUDZWA N. | South Africa

EIGHT

PULSELESS

> Good thing time isn't real and we're all going to die
> *Anonymous*

Dealing with death is an inevitable part of medical training. For many, the anatomy lab is usually the first introduction. For others, experiences from their own personal lives bring them to terms with death. In this chapter, trainees reflect on their experiences with death and the questions that surface from them.

Rigor Mortis

I saw a man once
Stare at me
On this ward.
He was dying
His lips were moving
But I couldn't hear him.
I think he wanted to talk to me
Speak Forty-Seven years of wisdom into my naivety.
I wonder if he was happy

If he lived right
If he has any regrets.
I wonder if he wanted to time-travel
Go back to the past
Unmake decisions
Or have a peep
Into a future he will never be a part of.
I wonder if he died a scared man
Unsure
Uncertain still
Of the life after this life
As the stiffness of rigor mortis kicked in.

AFOLABI B. | Nigeria

Shadow of Death

This is my first blog post as a first-year medical student. I had been debating whether to keep up the blog, but I figure, much like with teaching, the experiences that lie ahead of me will require reflection. So I guess here goes blogging part two:

Picking a field in medicine is akin to picking a major in college. You come into medical school having some general (or vague, or none, for that matter) idea of what you want to do. And like college, there are a ton of student groups that help foster that interest. For me, one possible career path has been emergency medicine (EM); so I joined the EM interest group. Students can also shadow in the ER. So tonight, I showed up for my first shadowing experience as a medical student.

At first, everything was going along pretty well. There were a lot of references to things that have come up in my classes that made the shadowing more worthwhile than when I was a very lost undergrad! I saw a central line get placed and my attending discussed a mnemonic for locating arteries and veins (something we'd just gone over today in our clinical skills group). I got to see the attending interview a patient and listen to his chest and review what parts of the lung could be heard. I saw some lab results of a patient with elevated CO_2 and the resulting effect on their blood pH; overheard that the radiologist found what they thought was a tumor on another patient's lingula and actually knew what a lingula was!

And then I saw the flurry of activity when the ER was informed that a "Trauma-1" was on the way. The paramedics arrived, administering CPR to the unresponsive person lying on the stretcher. Doctors and nurses, with stickers to denote their specialized role during the code, surrounded the patient. I stood as far back and out of the way as possible. One person was switched out for another to continue CPR compressions, but soon it was obvious that there was no pulse without them. And I heard them pronounce the death.

And. Just. Like. That . . . this person was gone.

I am pretty sure somewhere inside, a piece of me felt broken. To have been a bystander and see life slip away like a silk ribbon. It was devastating. All of it seemed so wrong, for someone to be there and then . . . not. I followed my attending out with tears building in my eyes. I was not surprised to see the pace return to pre-trauma levels rather quickly. The disappointed, but dry, faces of the staff were not unexpected either. My attending talked about the fact that while time doesn't make death easy, it does make dealing with death less hard.

As my tears dried and we checked on other patients from before, I thought I had shaken off the specter of the trauma code. But a while later, we piled into a corner room, and I listened to the resident deliver to a man an account of events that ended with, "Your wife has passed. She has died." This man had only been aware that his wife had been brought to the ER. The man I saw whole when we entered, I now saw broken, breaking, his face crumpling with searing emotion. I saw the moment of realization cross his face, as he shook his head trying not to believe what he had just heard. I saw the moment his tears joined the ones I'd been shedding in the corner. It was scary that as a doctor, you get to be part of these tragic, personal disasters.

The memory of his face when the news hit is still with me. The attending I shadowed said perhaps it would be a good thing if I never forgot it, that maybe when I did, I'd stop remembering why it was I wanted to be a doctor.

tammi c. | United States

Death and the Intern Experience

My senior resident turned to me: "You go pronounce him."

"*Me?*" But of course, that isn't what I said. That is never what you say as an intern. I peered through the glass into the patient room. His wife was leaning over his body, tears pouring down her face. She clutched his chest, then reached and closed his eyes with her hand. I took a deep breath and pulled back the curtain to the room. Five sets of tearful eyes looked up at me from bodies clothed in yellow gowns and gloves. The barriers now seemed odd in the moment.

"I am so sorry for your loss."

The words felt profoundly inadequate. I felt like an interloper caught in a moment that wasn't mine to experience. There were family members who couldn't make it in time and yet, I, a stranger, had been there. The family moved aside as I crossed the room toward the bed. I pulled back the blanket gingerly, exposing his gown. His chest was still warm. I did my post-mortem exam as the family looked on, muffled sobs surrounding me. I looked at the clock then looked at his wife and nodded. She nodded back. And that was it.

"What now?" they asked. What now indeed. "You can stay as long as you would like," I told them. They hugged and thanked me for everything. Thanked me? As his wife turned back to his body and began to sob, I turned and walked to the doorway, removed my yellow gown and blue gloves and pulled back the curtain. Outside of the room, a cacophony of sounds emerged: chatter, laughter, television shows in the next room, the beeps of monitors and the whirs of ventilators and hemodialysis machines. I walked briskly to the workroom to regain my composure. My computer screen blurred in front of me as I sat. I thought about my newborn son at home. My husband. My family. I was keenly aware that this moment wasn't about me, but it felt wrong not to mourn this family's loss.

His nurse peered in at me as I wiped away tears. She paused for a moment and studied my face. Just briefly. "You need to ask them if they want an autopsy," she offered, her face stoic, as she handed me the death certificate, explaining with it all of the ways I could mess things up if I didn't do it just right. It all felt too methodical. Too cold. But I did what I was told.

I watched as his wife walked away from the patient room. She hadn't left his side for more than a couple of minutes since the day he was admitted eight days prior. She hadn't left her husband's side for more than a couple of days in all thirty-five years of their marriage. Yet, she would now leave him behind in that hospital bed. Like clockwork, the hospitality cart outside of his room was wheeled away and his body was prepared for transport to the morgue.

As I headed out at the end of my night shift, I walked past his room. It was clean and sterile, bed empty, ready for the next patient. "Strong work today," a nurse called out as I walked out of the icu's double doors. I smiled, nodding weakly in response. Ahead, a group of nurses rolled a ventilated patient on a stretcher in my direction. The empty room would not be empty for long.

MARIAH R. | United States

Your Feet Were Cold As Ice

Your face is the last thing I see
every night before I go to sleep.
And the first thing I think of,
before my day begins.
There's no romance here. Or love.
Just worry. And fear.

You walked in on a Thursday morning.
And like how most love stories begin,
I had no idea my life
would be changed by having met you.

You stopped breathing.
And I think I did too.
Your heart stopped,
and mine might just have too.

The abscess weighed too heavily on your lung.
And I pumped, and I pumped, and I pumped
your chest to wake your heart.

But you stopped.
Pupils fixed. Asystole.

A woman came in
and I saw her whole life shatter.

Your feet were cold as ice.

MBULELO K. | South Africa

Nails

On a tired morning,
thoughts blurred by transition
between slumber and latte,
they welcome us to the brachial plexus.

Lost in the cables,
intrinsics and extrinsics,
I tune out
and find myself removing the moist glove.
But I'm jarred awake when I see
scarlet fingernails
stabbing the still laboratory air
in stiff rigor mortis.

I wonder:
What compelled her
to paint her nails red on that day?
Was it her favorite color
or was that just what she had around?

After a parade of strange faces and misdiagnoses,
after hours in ERS, ORS, and ICUS,
after fighting her own body for years,
were her nails her weapon?

A flag raised, not in surrender, but in defiance?
A middle finger to a distending aorta sewn together by
    titanium threads;
To bones made brittle by years of heavy mileage;
To a stuttering heart that beat with the eagerness of a
    crowning sun challenging the dawn?

I see her upturned fingers
pointing,
as if gesturing to Death,
"You want me?
Come and take me."

And I suppose he did.

But all I was given
were the words,
"myocardial infarction,"
written in black
next to my table number.

So I feel the need to fill in the blanks:
Shared cigarettes with long lost lovers;
Atherosclerotic coca-colas chilling frayed nerves;
One too many cocktails on a forgotten night with old friends.
I begin to see the factors that caused her death
as evidence that she was once alive.

Despite best efforts at de-identification,
these bonfire nails had somehow
slipped through the cracks.
Loud,
fiery,
stubborn,
red.

Why?

Maybe it was her message
to me, the student,
a cog in the medical machine
that had processed her.

To wake up
from the latte haze
and paint my life scarlet
while I still could.

samuel b. | United States

My Work of Breathing

7:53 P.M.
Thoughts of driving straight home run through my mind, punctuated by the familiar anxiety-inducing, high-pitched version of roadrunner emanating from my holstered pager.
Beep-beep, beep-beep
"Ms. X has passed. Please come pronounce. Thanks."
My head directs my eyes to roll because the universe has shown again, her commitment to ensuring that my luck stays unfortunate. My heart pangs wistfully because I got to know her a bit and did not expect it this early. I heave a sigh of acceptance and stand up, electing to get this over sooner rather than later. Resolve in hand, I run up the three flights of stairs it takes to accomplish my job. I arrive puffing, so I take a few seconds to catch a righting breath. I knock on the door and walk through. On the other side, staring at me are about eight expressions of grief, ranging from wistful smiles to active tears from bloodshot eyes. "Hello everyone, my name is Dr. Y."
I introduce myself and explain what I had come to do. Some faces nod in response. I walk over to pronounce, as I had been taught. I place my all-knowing stethoscope, and in that moment, I realize how quiet the room is. And because of this, I sense the intruding pound of tachycardia. My tachycardia. Since my heart is racing, asking for oxygen, I am forced to take a couple of pants as I get though the rest of the examination. When I finish, I turn back to the staring faces and give my condolences.

"I am so sorry for your loss."

"Thank you very much, Doctor," two or three voices reply as I walk out.

You know, it was not lost on me — the irony in having to catch my breath and satisfy my burning lungs to confirm that another's have ceased; the twisted mockery in feeling my bounding pulse to officially note the end of another's. I stood still and let the realization wash over me. Just long enough to allow the tears to start forming. Because in a minute, my head would take over and my new goal would be to get home. I closed my eyes and took in a restoring breath, deep enough to straighten my back and shoulders. When I opened my eyes back up, I let out a cleansing exhale. Then my head took over.

MOFIYIN O. | United States

Autopsy

We met, was it just the other day?
'Twas the middle of the night, when you came my way.
The emergency room transfer, to the medicine floor,
And my taking of your history, nearly sunrise, at four.

Your body had seen much, over decades of life spanned.
As an attorney and a husband, before life dealt you this
    hand.
Amyloid had ridden your organs, your heart most of all.
Ascites, kidney failure, and fibrillations, a heart nearing its last
    straw.

We spoke about the Capital,
Maryland crabs enriched with Old Bay.
And chuckled at the hospital-made eggs before you,
No savory seasoning had they.

And when I returned one morning,
In your bed, you were not there.
The night had turned your breath,
Into nothing else but air.

Not much later, I came to see you,
Though many floors below.
Your skin was cold and ashen,
A tag hung on your toe.

A heart that had loyally pumped,
For over a billion beats,
Lay still within my hands,
Your other organs lain in sheets.

As I held your enlarged heart,
Nearly twice the normal being's,
I had a rush of insatiable thoughts,
About what the body truly means.

Our medical questions had been answered
After seeing your insides out.
But as I held your heart,
I could not help but incur doubt.

Are we really all just capsules?
Is this really it?
Once breath and spirit leave the body,
Alone our capsules sit.
I know not what comes after life,
If there is anything more.
Autopsies show us many things.
Though the soul's fate, we implore.

FAITH R. | United States

The Red Line

"Time of death—9:13 a.m."

I was standing behind the red line in the trauma bay, the marking an arbitrary delineation to somehow make us feel removed from the organized chaos that was usually happening on the other side of it. I didn't feel very removed from it that morning.

The end of a twenty-nine-hour shift was quickly approaching. I had thankfully caught my second wind early in the morning, finally able to do something useful with my fourth-year medical student status as I hastily prepared the patient lists for morning sign out. The residents were downstairs tending to the twelfth trauma of the night shift. I worked through the lists quickly. Vitals. Ins and outs. New labs. Check. On to the next patient and repeat. I made copies and left for the elevator, stopping along the way to look outside the tenth floor window at the ending sunrise, feeling content in the moment.

Morning sign out started at 8:30 a.m. for the teams to go through the list of patient updates. It was towards the end of it that another trauma came in—a gunshot wound. As the day shift residents rushed downstairs to the trauma bay, I stayed upstairs with the night shift team to finish sign out. It was a last-minute decision that I decided to go downstairs just to watch.

There were more people than usual crowded behind the red line. It was quiet, which is something I still find myself occasionally surprised by. Most people picture the loud chaos that is often presented in television shows, but in reality, it's not like that. Quiet is needed to yell out what is happening with the patient—orders and physical exam findings and IV access success are shouted out in a systematic fashion. My job as a medical student during a trauma is to silently cut off patients' clothes and cover them with warm blankets—to cover up their dignity as I also ironically cut away the only thing they come into the hospital with. Up until then, the patients I had seen had come in stable, but this time I walked up to something quite different.

A cracked open chest. Blood spilled on the floor. Extensive resuscitative measures. The attending's hands shoved into the patient's chest, around his heart, desperately searching for the injury. It was found. A bullet through the heart. An injury that can't be survived. Everyone stopped what they were doing, and time of death was called.

9:13 a.m.

I could see the patient's feet poking through the blankets they were covered with, already looking paler. There was a part of me that wanted to reach out to touch his toes just to see if they were already going cold from lack of blood flow.

The trauma attending took time after that to teach. After all, it wasn't every day that there was fresh anatomy splayed open and available like it was. He explained the difference in feel between the esophagus and the aorta. The former has a gritty feel, the latter does not. There was a part of me that was initially outraged at the objective coldness of what was occurring. The patient had just died in a horrible fashion. What were his family or friends thinking, if he even had any? Were they picturing us doing everything we could to save their family member? Although that had indeed been done, I wondered what they would have thought about us doing an advanced anatomy lesson so quickly afterwards? The patient's toes may have started going cold, but certainly there were still parts that were warm. But then I looked at it from a different standpoint. What he was teaching would save more lives in the future, in an emergent situation where perhaps the only thing to rely on to save life was not imaging, fancy equipment, or even visual inspection, but rather, a blind feel to identify a major injury—the gritty versus the smooth.

Still not sure how to feel, I gowned up and stepped forward past the red line to learn. The first thing I noticed were the black specks on the patient's lungs—evidence of a smoking history. *Inspection, check.* I looked at the attending and asked if he could show me. He nodded and began. I indeed felt the difference between the gritty esophagus and the smooth aorta. Next, I moved to the heart. Still warm. How about the toes? One of my fingers soon moved through the back of the heart as another moved through the front. They met in the middle in a way that they should never have been able to, had a bullet not carved a path through the tissue. *Palpation, check.*

As the heart was no longer beating and the lungs no longer breathing, auscultation could not be performed. Not wanting to linger, I moved back behind the red line. I contemplated what to do next and the first thought that popped into my head was whether to go eat breakfast right then or to wait until I got home. The thought came before I could stop it and I immediately felt shame crawl through me. Then I felt torn over whether I should even be burdened by shame for thinking of eating right after what had happened. I struggle a lot these days with the concept of humanity in medicine, especially in the field of surgery. How can one maintain their sense of humanism and vulnerability and emotional connection when one is constantly subjected to seeing difficult and emotionally impactful things on a constant basis? Is there a way to healthily disconnect? It's something I fear for myself, and thinking of whether to eat breakfast or not brought that fear up immediately.

I thought back to earlier in the evening when another patient had arrived with a knife broken off in the back of his neck after being stabbed. The patient arrived miraculously stable, but nobody initially knew if the knife was embedded in any major blood vessels. As the team worked to make that determination, the patient was lying motionless on the trauma bed so as not to disturb the knife. He was fully coherent, though his speech was soft and mumbled. I remember leaning down as close as possible to gather his medical information. I wondered whether he thought he was going to die. He must have. Death had been a very real possibility, but thankfully his toes were still warm. The only sign that betrayed his knowledge of the severity of the situation were the tears rolling down his face. As he answered my questions he was unable to reach up and wipe them away. I grabbed a tissue and spent a moment dabbing at his tears and holding his hand in silence. It was the only thing I could do. I had a thought that wiping his tears was equally as important as any question I had asked. Because what is medicine if humanity is absent?

Thankfully, the knife had missed anything important and it was safely pulled out in the OR without any further issues. However, we did discover later that the patient had stage four lung cancer. The irony was not lost on me—saved by external forces only to undoubtedly succumb to internal forces in what would probably be a few months.

I went home that morning with thoughts of these two stories heavy on my mind, both humbling examples of how human connection is inseparable from every patient we encounter. I also went home unsure of how to feel, but I did know that I was disturbed and scared of what the future was going to hold. Would I be able to find a balance? How much should I remove my emotions from a situation, not just to protect myself, but also to protect a patient from the fact that emotions can skew a logical decision? Is there a healthy way to do it? How do the residents I have watched during trauma calls cope? Can I handle this? Am I strong enough?

I don't have answers to any of these questions, and I don't think I will soon—at least not without a few more years of experience. However, I can imagine that the questions never truly end. Either way, the fine balance between disconnecting and connecting is something I desperately hope to maintain the correct perspective on. Right now, the most I can do is to keep striving to be the doctor—and the person—that I want to be . . . one that doesn't forget the value of human connection and its intrinsic link with medicine.

CHRISTINA G. | United States

Eyelashes

The boy had skeletal arms, skin stretched tight over protruding ribs, and a balloon belly like a comical fat suit. I was working at a rural hospital in northern Ghana for the month. The rotation fulfilled my medical school's rural family medicine clerkship requirement, but in truth, it was an intense mishmash of internal medicine, pediatrics, obstetrics, surgery, and all the associated subspecialties.

During my time there, the boy visited the hospital frequently for paracenteses. The first time we met, his ascitic fluid was thick and bloody—watered-down tomato juice. He remained inflated despite three litres drained, but we were able to palpate the rough nodular surface, the crannies—the mountainous landscape of his liver that extended far beyond the normal margins. Hepatocellular cancer (HCC) had anchored his insides.

He lay stoic as the peritoneal fluid flowed. His eyes were wide and almond shaped, exaggerated by his thinness. His eyelashes curled 360 degrees on themselves. With high angular cheekbones, plump round lips, and the delay of puberty that often comes with chronic disease, he was delicate and pixie-like. Initially, the paracentesis improved his symptoms, but several days later he returned for another fix. Again we drained it. Again it was bloody. This time he winced as we stuck him with the needle. I expected his belly to deflate, a popped balloon.

The following week, he reappeared moaning in pain, legs edematous, belly beyond comical. Farcical. Unreal. Unfair. The boy was singing a soft wail that pierced my ears and twisted my bowels until I felt queasy. The staff physician had decided it futile—unsustainable—to continue the taps. The boy's father was at his side. His mother had shed a single tear the day prior, before hurriedly wiping it away. Otherwise, they were calm.

Lost in my own questions about paracenteses and its utility in HCC, about pain and palliative medications and potential next steps, I didn't notice his whimpering soften. There were no breath sounds when I pushed my stethoscope into his back or when I balanced it on his bony ribs. His chest was still. My face inches from his. I ran my index finger over his eyelashes like a comb. No blink. I pressed the fleshy part of my fingers into his wrist. *Was that a heartbeat? I swear I felt a pulse.* But nothing was beating. When I listened over his heart, silence. I had felt my own pulse, not his, my own life source flowing through him and back to me. I waited and watched; not the full, painful five or ten minutes we do at home, but about two or three. He had no blink reflex, no obvious last gasp, no heartbeat, no final wail of pain, just an unnoted slide into death and silence. And seconds later from outside in the hall, his mother cried the scream he couldn't produce: the howl of pain and irreplaceable love and loss, of regret and anger and bitter, bitter agony.

I was arrested by my role as a student and a visitor in a socio-medical culture vastly different from my own. Concerned about my role as a potential neo-colonizer, I was hypersensitive to the complex ties engendered in these interactions. The fear of doing the wrong thing was paralyzing. Yet in the space of contemplation and inaction, not only did I fail to provide a soft transition into death, I let the patient-physician bond fall to the wayside.

As medical students and physicians, we become part of our patients' stories, of how they live and how they die. We build the scaffolding upon which patients and families can string coherent narratives of "the circle of life." And that is what ultimately gives life, and death, meaning. We might be powerless to change the final outcome, but can change the journey. While contemplating the boy's next best medical step, I lost the person in front of me. The scaffolding lay half-constructed and limp, unable to withstand the weight of his unachieved hopes, unable to support the weight of his parents' loss. I was wracked with guilt. But guilt stymies, it doesn't incite positive action. Since then, I have made a strong commitment to listening to my patients, to really hearing them, and to recognizing that inaction may be as—if not more—injurious than making the wrong decision. I won't ever forget those eyelashes.

MAXIME B. | Canada

Preparing for Death

I walked dutifully into Richard's room to conduct a full history and physical, and stopped in the doorway. The buzzing, off-white light illuminated the soft glow of his yellow skin. His eyes remained shut and his family's eyes darted to mine, sensing my apprehension. Richard likely had an obstruction in his biliary tract system, and I was most worried that he had terminal cancer because of his age (seventy-one years old) and abrupt overall decline. "All of a sudden he stopped eating and wouldn't talk to anyone," Richard's wife anxiously offered as I took the admission history. "It's as if Richard vanished—I was so scared," she continued.

"Two weeks ago, he was telling jokes at dinner with the whole family. We couldn't stop laughing!" Richard's oldest daughter reminisced. "We went for walks every week, up until last Wednesday. I know he has dementia but this all happened . . . so quickly," she added softly, her eyes trailing back to her father.

Despite the dim light, his jaundiced face contrasted with his gray, straight hair. "Richard, can you tell me where you are right now?" I asked, gently. Richard's family stared at him, waiting patiently until he broke the silence after what seemed like an eternity. "B—O—S—T—O—N," Richard replied exceedingly slowly, struggling with each syllable. His eyes tracked to mine, but he could not engage with me.

This was the most Richard would speak now, and he barely responded to me with one-word answers, eventually only moaning in pain and breathing rapidly. Our team's efforts needed to focus on allowing Richard and his family to understand his poor prognosis and, most importantly, that the end was near. Over the last few weeks, none of his doctors had prepared Richard or his family, and now it was up to me. Each day, our medical team would round outside Richard's room, peering in to see a warm crowd surrounding him. I would update his daughter, the family's spokesperson, who was hopeful, but the facts remained that he was getting worse.

I was scared when I first saw Richard. When we met, my mind flashed back to ten years earlier, when my then fifty-five-year-old father was about to undergo bypass heart surgery—a major operation. At the time, I had no reason to believe my father wouldn't make a good recovery. I knew he needed a serious procedure, but his doctors thought he would recuperate well given his relatively young age. One month later, in the middle of the night, I would find my *Abba*—Hebrew for dad—lifeless in his bed. My mother woke me after she found him there. I desperately called 911 and within minutes, EMS personnel were carrying my father into an ambulance.

The fear of Richard's impending death startled me. Years earlier, I lost my father, and I became a physician, partly, to help stave off death. But here I was, watching an elderly man die in front of me, surrounded by the immense love of his family. I had known logically since the start of my training that I would experience death again as a doctor, but the wave of helplessness in this moment shook me more than I had anticipated.

Richard continued to spike high fevers despite antibiotics, and moaned occasionally, unable to follow commands or open his eyes.

Richard was dying, and I felt responsible for helping to prepare his family for the worst. Yet, I also resisted admitting that this was to be my project, my role. For years, I had worked to become a physician to heal people—to give people new time with dying loved ones—time that I did not have when I found my own father ten years earlier.

In a large family discussion with Richard's primary medical team and liver and kidney specialists, we spoke about Richard's poor prognosis. "His kidneys are shutting down. The fevers suggest that he has an infection in his body—most likely in his gastrointestinal tract, and his mental status has not improved. I am worried we are heading in the wrong direction," I said directly. "What would your father want?" I inquired further, thinking about the many times I've posed this incredible question to families. I thought about never having heard this question posed to my father before his surgery—my family never had this discussion.

"He would never want to live like this—suffering and feeling so helpless," Richard's daughter jumped in. "We talked about this only a month ago on one of our walks through the park. 'When it's time, let me go. I've told enough jokes this lifetime,' he said to me. I hate seeing him like this," she cried to me. Richard's wife looked deeply into her dear husband's empty, yellow eyes. Richard's family understood he likely had cancer but was too sick to undergo invasive, definitive testing. With each passing day, his family prepared more for his death; as did I, knowing I could not save him either. Together, Richard's family agreed to decline extreme measures: if he were to stop breathing or if his heart were to stop beating, there would be no chest compressions or intubation ("DNR/DNI"), and we would pursue comfort measures only ("CMO") and allow for the natural course of his disease, as he had wished.

During this time, I found myself thinking routinely about my father. A few days after his major surgery. I walked into his bare white room after work—I had a summer internship in a local bank's IT department after my freshman year. My dad's soft grayish skin contrasted sharply with the bright red heart-shaped pillow he hugged—I later learned this pillow was part of the standard post-operative recovery process.

"Amir—how—was—work?" My dad asked, casually, taking slow, deep breaths in between his words. He winced with each breath, clutching his pillow harder. The nasal cannula was only in one of his nostrils—I reached over to adjust it. Multiple catheters pumped fluids and medicines directly into his veins; he could barely move without a new alarm sounding. "*Abba*, it was awesome—I got to rebuild and set up a whole office of computers at one of the branches!" I said excitedly, knowing my dad wanted to hear more. "We got the new Intel motherboards and memory. I know the tellers will appreciate the upgrade," I added. "Whoa, how cool! Now we can upgrade my office computer in the basement," My dad responded eagerly, pushing through the rib pain. He was an engineer and loved to take me to the local computer show to see the new equipment and upgrade our systems. His nurse had said he was recovering well and could return home in another day. I left eager to go to work the next day—to learn how to install a hard drive and video card on the new workstations. I wanted to build a supercomputer with my dad when he returned home.

One afternoon my pager beeped, "Richard expired. Please come pronounce." I sprinted downstairs, gently knocking on the door, and walked in. His entire family filled the dark and somber room. There was a fruit basket and pastries next to a book about grieving. Richard's wife was by his side, crying in silence and clutching her fists. Richard's body lay lifeless in bed; I stood beside him as if it were ten years earlier, when the doctors from the hospital told my mother and me that my father was gone. My father had suffered a fatal heart attack one month after his supposed lifesaving surgery. Richard died, likely of an infection as a complication of a terminal cancer, losing an internal battle.

I left that day torn between feeling as if I had helped, and as if I had not. I wanted nothing more than to help Richard, but all I did was facilitate his passing. For Richard's family, pursuing comfort measures reflected their preparation for his death, knowing he would not want to suffer any longer and to die peacefully. I wanted to make sure Richard was comfortable, something I wondered if my father felt on that night ten years ago. As the doctor now, I wanted nothing more than to help Richard's family get through this experience, as the doctors helped my family; I also wanted to help Richard's family in ways those doctors had not. I was confronted with a patient I could not save; I was confronted with a situation that made me wonder how much of my own path to medical school was motivated by an effort to grapple with death as that which is both deeply human and beyond human control. I knew, in helping Richard and his family, that there was never a way for a person to have a "good" death, whether sudden or not. And yet I worked to prepare Richard's family as best I could, wishing I had had someone to prepare me for the harsh finality of losing my father so abruptly.

Although medical advances allow patients to live longer, they still are sicker and may die more gradually—with a lower quality of life than perhaps expected. As physicians, we need to discuss death more openly. All physicians, regardless of specialty, should feel empowered to have these discussions with their patients, especially as patients cope with grave diagnoses. Throughout my medical training, I learned the intricacies of the human body and disease—but never have I been taught how to prepare for when my patient's body is failing and nearing death. The intricacies of familial emotions surrounding death will always be a lifelong learning process, but as gatekeepers for the human body, physicians must learn to openly discuss the reality of death with our patients and families—to help others to process and understand it to the best of their ability. I also believe that risk of death should be discussed more openly between physicians and patients. I wish my father's surgeons spoke to my family and me about the very real fatal complications after such a significant operation. Discussing death in the context of serious diagnoses more openly may help patients and their families better prepare for the realities they face.

Support is what was offered to me ten years ago, though it felt inadequate and too late. Today, I still struggle with how my family and I could have prepared for my dad's death. And

I wonder if the doctors I interacted with ten years earlier could have helped more. All I know is no one prepared me enough — and I am also aware that a piece of me understands in a new way that no one ever could.

AMIR M. | United States

NINE

PRODIGAL

I need to run off this existential crisis.

Anonymous

People chart different courses in medicine. Some courses are fairly linear, others are labyrinthine, complete with elaborate detours. These detours themselves can take on many forms, whether it's taking time off to raise a child or getting a second degree. Sometimes even, a trainee decides to leave medicine altogether. In this chapter trainees speak of their forays outside medicine and tell of how they are learning to navigate the worlds they straddle.

Code Switch

This time last year,
MD meant only one thing.
But since then, I have frolicked
in the world of balance sheets and shareholders,
exchanged patients for customers,
and swapped treatment plans for org strategy.

MD now means two things for me,
and I must learn to switch seamlessly
between the two.

TOLU K. | United States

Dr. Wife to Mrs. Mom

I recently quit my job. And by job, I mean residency. As those
in the field can attest, this isn't something that happens often.
Once you start, it's expected that you'll finish, regardless of how
difficult things get, no matter the sacrifice. Online forums advise
residents considering leaving to "forget about it," cautioning that
leaving is not worth it after everything one goes through to get
to, and go through, residency.

And they're right about how much goes into medicine. I went
through four years of undergraduate training, endured countless
hours of studying for classes like Organic Chemistry and Phys-
ics, and slaved away doing research in dark basement laborato-
ries. I stood on my feet for endless hours, shadowing attending
physicians like an imprinted baby duck; studied for, and took
the hours-long MCAT. I spent thousands of dollars flying around
the country for medical school interviews. Then, once in medical school, I suffered through exam after exam, spent hours on
end dissecting dead bodies, again stood on my feet endlessly
as we rounded on rotation after rotation, all the while playing
"yes man (or woman)" to my seniors. I studied for Steps one &
two, and again spent thousands of dollars on flights around the
country interviewing for residency. So why would I, who regu-
larly tried to skip recess in elementary school to do work and
get ahead, decide to give it all up? My family.

Before applying to medical school, I said a prayer that if God
wanted me to go to medical school, He would make a way for
my future family to be a priority. I had actually forgotten about

this prayer along the way, but throughout med school, God always did exactly that. Sometimes, He would place me with the right senior residents. Other times, He would place me on a schedule that allowed me to leave the hospital at a decent time. One time, He even provided the time for me to get married during medical school. This time, however, God reminded me of my prayer and I felt like He was calling me to step out in faith and continue to make my family a priority. When our baby boy showed up, I knew I had to make a decision.

As a resident, days are long, with most work weeks fluctuating between sixty–eighty hours. In the beginning, our little one was usually sound asleep when I left for work, and I would get home with just enough time to shower, feed him, and put him to sleep. I envisioned the next four years with me missing his first words and steps, missing his first taste test of solid food and his first Christmas—I wouldn't be ok with that. God had blessed me with this special gift and I knew that putting him on the back burner while I pursued my career wasn't an option for me. After all, there would always be more doctors, but only one person who would be Micah's mom.

I get questions from people who think I've wasted all my prior efforts. I have my thoughts on why God blessed me with such an extensive education, and I believe in the future He will provide other ways for me to use it. People also ask if I'll ever return to medicine. Thankfully, my institution provided me the unusual option to return if I later felt so inclined. I don't know what the future holds, or if I will return, but for right now, I know what I need to do.

*This piece was originally published on www.mrsmomdrwife.com

SHEREE B. | United States

Returning to Once Familiar Territory

Although four years might seem like a lengthy time in medical school, the experience is incredibly fast-paced. Sequentially focusing on one organ system to the next, covering topics ranging from anatomy to pathology, the first two years of medical school provide a necessarily condensed introduction to the entirety of medicine. At the start of third year, the transition out of the classroom and into the hospital happens almost too quickly.

For the minority of MD students that additionally pursue a basic science PhD, the rapid pace of medical training is entirely redirected. Instead of being funneled from the classroom and into the hospital environment, aspiring physician-scientists like myself experience a major deceleration. Clinical training is paused while we plunge into an expansive and dynamic world of basic research.

TIME-LAPSE EDUCATION

After five years of deep devotion to the biology underlying brain development, I finally returned to medical school. Even for an experienced bench scientist with formidable laboratory skills, I had hesitations. Yes, my research was clinically motivated, but it was a long time apart from clinical thinking. And there had been significant changes in that time. When I paused my medical training five years ago, smartphones were in their infancy, and their utility in medicine, entirely unanticipated. I am amused by my classmates' replacement of penlights with iPhones, and the juxtaposition of their speedy iPad apps to my outdated medical books. Five years ago, my professors never emphasized today's popular clinical topics, including the risks of X-ray imaging, the spiraling costs of healthcare, or the increasing concerns over health information privacy. In addition, recent work-hour restrictions have markedly changed the tone and tempo of the clinical environment.

To add to the unfamiliarity of my reentry to medicine, my medical school adopted curriculum changes that significantly restricted the flexibility of my upcoming third and fourth years in medical school. Even my MD/PhD program replaced its leadership twice, leaving me out of touch with my current director. After five short years, both my school and the medical field seemed more distant than I could have expected.

"BETTER TO HAVE LEARNED IT ONCE . . ."

Five years is also a long time to forget some clinical basics. One of the first patients I saw as a third-year medical student had a skin infection. After I gave a thoughtful bedside presentation, my attending asked me, "What are the common causes of skin infections?" "What classes of antibiotics cover these types of bacteria?" "How do these antibiotics function?" I stumbled on each question. My preceptor was aghast. How could a third-year medical student not answer these relatively straightforward questions? Although my well-intentioned preceptor had never worked with a post-PhD medical student, he was visibly concerned about my ability to succeed this year. I quietly recalled my pathology professor from six years ago who had proclaimed, "Better to have learned it once, than to have never learned it." Back then I worked hard to master the answers to these kinds of questions. Unfortunately, the payoff will have to wait for some future time.

PERSONAL GROWTH

Although it is easier to comment on the many changes in my clinical environment, I too have changed. I'm now married. I have new nephews and in-laws. My siblings have moved on with their lives and careers. I have successfully navigated through a relatively intense and stressful PhD experience. These factors combined, I feel more resilient to the small stresses of clinical training.

Alongside these personal developments, my professional outlook and priorities have sharpened. In contrast to the distinct and protected time of my first two years of medical school and then my PhD, this phase of my training now incorporates both clinical and research responsibilities. By necessity, I have adjusted my time management to simultaneously catch up on medicine, finish research manuscripts, and explore viable residency options. With increasing focus, I am beginning to navigate the professional challenges of a physician-scientist.

THE FAMILIAR SIDE OF MEDICINE

Despite the different nature of my clinical experiences after a five-year hiatus, some core experiences in medicine are unchanged. Last month, I evaluated a healthy fifty-year-old gentleman on a routine physical. He didn't initially complain of chest pain, but during my exam, I identified very mild symptoms that were concerning for possible angina. My attending and I referred him to appropriate diagnostic testing, and over a few short days, he was given the unexpected diagnosis of major coronary artery disease that required urgent bypass surgery. Contributing to the early identification of this life-threatening condition has been one of my most gratifying clinical experiences to date, and one that reminds me of what I love about medicine.

Looking forward, I hope to continue adapting to the ongoing and unpredictable challenges of being a young physician-scientist. While the scientific world will undoubtedly mature and change during my present clinical training, I wonder if a future return to the laboratory will be as unfamiliar as my present return to the clinic. At that unknown time, I hope I find myself to be a resilient player who finds familiar territory despite changing actors, tools, and opportunities.

CAMERON S. | United States

TEN

ADULT DREAMS

An odd ratio
of human and machine,
I am slowly becoming.
Trevor M.

*Time is an asset, one that changes your perspectives and provides
you with a wealth of experiences to formulate opinions on. In this
closing chapter, trainees reflect on how both they and their interests
have changed over time. Based on a time-enhanced, nuanced view
of the medicine, they also speak out on aspects of the medicine they
would like to see change.*

(Un)twisted

Is it a crime to love,
Love what I do, love who I have become?
I feel like a prisoner to the choices I have made.
I feel guilt for the sacrifices I have made to become a healer;
Questioning the decisions that have brought me from one
    eight-hour exam to the next.

I refuse to glorify suffering,
To pride in meaningless work devoid of true satisfaction.
I refuse to measure my work by how many uninterrupted
  hours I spend at the hospital.
I refuse to feel guilt for choosing,
Choosing to love my life, love what I do, love who I am and
  who I will become

I will pride in my choices to become a healer,
A healer that rises above the culture of senseless martyrdom,
Above the systems that oppress and overlook the humanity of
  the healer.
I choose to enjoy my career in medicine.
I choose to say no to a twisted notion.

PEACE E. | United States

Wretch: Lost, Found, and Lost Again

It starts in a little rural hospital on the Thai-Burma border. I'm
sprawled on a concrete bench in the Emergency Department,
wrestling with the wording of my medical school application
essay. Without warning, a truck barrels into the ambulance bay.
I stash my notebook and help to pull a deeply feverish man onto
a rickety metal gurney. A young monk, Burmese by the deep
maroon of his robes, climbs from the back of the truck and hurries after us into the hospital's lone emergency room. There's a
flurry of activity. No one can find a BP, much less a decent vein.
I hold the patient's legs as Dr. Bo, a young Thai woman just
out of medical school, tries to insert an endotracheal tube. He
arches violently, vomiting a purulent-looking green substance
onto her sandals. She tries again, nails it, and he flails wildly
in protest—even if someone could start a line, Etomidate and
Sux are luxuries this hospital can't afford to waste. The monk,

who turns out to be a friend of the patient, hovers anxiously. The nurses deftly avoid contact; even in the middle of the chaotic scene, they bow their heads when they whisk by, take care not to brush against him inadvertently. The patient is wheeled off to the ICU, and the monk is left, bewildered, in the ER.

One of the male doctors is called in to deal with the monk. He speaks softly and respectfully through one of the Burmese orderlies, explaining about pneumonia and sepsis and tubes and antibiotics. The prognosis is not good, he says, but the care here is excellent. The doctor's sorrow for the other man's suffering is clear on his face. It seems to help.

I watch the scene unfold, feeling fevered myself. *This is Exciting. This is Useful. We are Helping People while Respecting Cultural and Personal Boundaries. We are Doing the Best We Can with Limited Resources. We are Being Kind.* This is exactly what I want to do for the rest of my life.

Med school: At orientation they told us to think of the four-year scramble to master the medical knowledge of the ages as "a marathon, not a sprint," ensured us that we'd soon be able to gulp facts like "water from a fire hose." They were right, in a way: we all, to varying degrees, adapted to the rigorous pace set by our faculty. We figured out how to sleep less and caffeinate more and immerse ourselves in a pool of anxiety and willpower so that we could process the material they cranked out. They left out, though, what we might lose in the process.

I'd never been that busy, that intensely tuned to a particular academic wavelength. There was the Krebs cycle and pressure-volume loops and clinical exam skills and all manner of things to memorize and master. Everything extraneous was abandoned. I didn't have the time or energy to think about the things I'd seen in Thailand, to talk with my classmates about all the suffering we were seeing in our clinical preceptors' offices, to understand what "medicine as a tool for social justice" meant now that I was a real-live medical student. We paused occasionally for a course called Professions of Medicine, where we discussed the "hidden curriculum" of medical school: how doctors learn to behave towards themselves, their colleagues, their patients; what it means to suffer as a patient, what it means as a doctor to watch this suffering. You know . . . emotional stuff. And then a roomful of exhausted, emotionally overwrought medical students would commence to cry in droves (while a significant portion pulled faces at how all of this soft stuff was a waste of time).

When winter break rolled around, I emerged from a study-driven stupor to find myself utterly drained. I was so physically exhausted that the little girl in the downstairs apartment startled when she saw my face. "Did someone punch you?" "No, dear-heart, that's just the bags under my eyes." I was an existential wreck as well: I didn't know how to navigate now that I was no longer the smartest person in the room. I was sick of the monotonous work. I was being nibbled to death by persistent questions that I had neither the time nor the emotional capacity to address.

Do I have any value to add in this context?

How do I keep myself intact given these time and ego pressures?

How do I learn the skills necessary for dealing with suffering (mine? My patients?)?

How, if at all, should I modulate my own values/beliefs/behaviors in response to the culture of medicine, which can be cruel?

Was I naive to think that I could make any real difference?

But I had a new project to work on, a fellowship inspired by the Schwartz Center for Compassionate Healthcare. I showed up at the first research meeting with an ill-formed question and no idea how to answer it: "Um. I'm interested in how medical students in other cultures learn compassion? Because I spent all this time with doctors in Thailand and they seemed exceedingly kind and dedicated and compassionate? And so maybe they're teaching their med students something that we can learn about and then do over here?" Pano Rodis (the same gentle soul who so carefully constructed our mass catharsis sessions) listened to me ramble, considered, and then suggested, "Why don't you work with Manish?" This was either extremely insightful or an excellent stroke of luck. Dr. Manish Mishra turned out to be a physician with a firm belief in "following one's questions." For someone with as many questions as I, this was an unspeakable relief.

At Manish's suggestion, I started off by trying to define compassion. After all those months of laser-like focus, I let myself fly off the handle a bit, throwing myself at the project with vigor, if not an excess of organization. I fell into a series of intellectual sinkholes: linguistic, anthropological, philological, etymological, historical. (What does it mean to define a word, a concept? From what intellectual framework does one even approach such a question?) I befriended the Dartmouth librarians and combed through PubMed for relevant publications. I watched Buddhist monks lecture, paged through the relevant bits of the New Testament, listened to Arjuna and Krishna chat till they were both blue in the face.

For reasons both practical and poetic, I chose to move my cross-cultural project to the back burner and decided to focus on physicians closer to home. Over the course of three months, I conducted twelve hour-long interviews with doctors at Dartmouth, asking about their understanding and practice of compassion. I was hoping to glean something teachable, something that could be implemented in the Dartmouth curriculum to help medical students like me grow into the sorts of doctors we came to medical school to be.

How do you define compassion?

Do you consider yourself a compassionate physician?

How can you tell when you're delivering compassionate care?

Can you tell me about a time when you didn't deliver compassionate care? Why did that happen?

Do you think compassion is teachable?

While I reveled in the opportunity to ask impertinent questions and soaked up wisdom from the physicians who so generously allowed themselves to be interviewed by a lowly first-year medical student, definitive answers to my questions were not forthcoming. I found that many doctors hadn't considered compassion in any serious way. Most physicians, when asked to define compassion, balked; an odd finding, given that they all claimed to consider themselves to be compassionate practitioners. None of the docs had a very clear idea about how compassion develops, but most believed that medical students tend to show up to medical school with compassionate values (even if they don't necessarily have the skills to put those values into practice). They spoke of models, both positive and negative, who had shown them (often inadvertently) what compassion does and does not look like. Some even spoke at length about Narrative Medicine, Leadership, and Resilience as methods to nurture, teach, and protect compassion. Many said that they wished they had more empirical evidence about whether or not the "compassionate" methods they employed were effective (in changing patient behavior, in altering emotional states in a positive and lasting way). Some docs spoke about the healthcare system as a whole, how its current focus on productivity and record keeping can require physicians to defer their compassionate impulses in order to accomplish the tasks required by their employers. They spoke of unkind teachers, impatient co-workers, and a desire to "join the club" of medical culture, even though they often found it to be cruel to doctors and patients alike.

I planned to spend my summer working through the interviews I'd collected, finding commonalities and pearls of insight, perhaps even transcribing and coding the responses to produce a set of quantitative data. I'd received a bit of grant money to conduct a chart review at the hospital in Thailand where I'd been before; I figured I'd work through the charts during the days and process my compassion data in the evenings and emerge from the summer triumphant. *But then I got to Thailand and everything got shot to hell.*

I'm sitting at the nurse's station, waiting for the doctors to show up for morning rounds. This ward smells of disinfectant and cooked vegetables and warm blood. The man two beds down on the right is dying. I can hear the rattle from here. His family has a cell phone to his ear, monks chanting Buddhist scripture in Pali. One of his relatives, a young guy about my age, has had his eye on me since I walked in. There's something about the tilt of his eyebrows, the dampness of his gaze; I see in his eyes that he thinks I might fix this, that by virtue of my white coat or my whiteness I can pull his father or uncle or grandfather from the maw of death. I am ashamed, deeply ashamed, of my uselessness. But I will not hide from him, will not shirk from the suffering directly in front of me. I swallow and meet his gaze. I can't speak to him — he's Karen, not Thai, and anyway I can barely choke this stuff out in my mother tongue — but I try to let this show on my face: "I see your suffering. I can't fix it. I am so, so, sorry." He gets it, his face modulates. We both look away.

I think back to the hours I spent interviewing nice, healthy physicians in tidy, affluent Hanover. I remember the hours spent carefully crafting and ordering Anthropologically Appropriate interview questions, the earnest practicing on peers, the pushing and cajoling and endearing to coax some candor out of folks I'd just met. I remember ironing my skirt and lining my eyes so that the Real Doctors would take me seriously, sitting in the clean offices where people sat around and thought about the patient experience all day, where the electricity never went off and the drugs never ran out. I can't remember why I did all that, why it seemed to matter at the time.

The next day, it is a tiny wrinkled woman who is vomiting blood in the dingy ER. "I can't breathe, I can't breathe," she whispers between heaves. "Please help me." The lab says it's scrub typhus; it often is. She's had a fever for two weeks, and her family is just now bringing her in. If she'd come in a week ago, it'd have been a different story, but they didn't, so here we are.

The doctor has had enough of this. "You! Are you her daughter? How much does she drink? No, I mean it, don't lie to me, how much does she drink?" She drinks a lot. The family is ashamed. Everyone in the outpatient waiting room can hear. "You need to find everyone you know and bring them here to donate plasma." The hospital doesn't have the facilities to store fresh frozen plasma (FFP)—it's expensive, and besides, when the electricity goes out five or ten times a day, you can hardly keep milk without it going bad. "What are you doing standing around? Don't you understand? She could die from this; do you understand that or not?" The daughter tears, nods, and leaves on her motorcycle to round up her family. The woman dies the next day anyway.

It's the unfairness of it all. The eminently preventable suffering. The uselessness of the pain. The placid acceptance of death and disease and disfigurement. The bright, shiny metal cylinders with bags of FFP nestled among the liquid nitrogen in bright, shiny New Hampshire. The Child Life Specialists and Tranquility Gardens and Grief Circles. The lidocaine, for crying out loud. When the disparities are this deep, how can I dedicate anything less than all of my resources to rectifying them? How can I justify my ivory tower compassion interviews?

A floppy yellow baby is pulled full-term and lifeless from his mother in an ambulance stuck on the muddy precipice of a cliff. He rides back to the hospital in a crisp plastic bag at his mother's feet. Is this compassion? Two drivers, two nurses, a doctor, and a random farang (white person) driving three hours into the jungle to try to save this woman and her baby. No charge. Risking life and limb and headlong crashes down the mountain. But there are no soft words spoken to the mother who has just lost her child. Nothing in particular said to the father, who has surely been at this project of giving birth for hours and hours, if not days. Here, there is sacrifice. There is effort. There is dedication to the cause of health. But is this loving-kindness, exactly? Is this compassion? Hard to know. Maybe I need to expand my definition.

I asked the Hanover physicians how they felt when their patients died, how they kept themselves open to caring while protecting themselves from emotional collapse. Who gives a crap? I asked these physicians to tell me the strategies they used to communicate compassion to their recalcitrantly obese/smoking/drinking/drugging patients. The $100 they charge for an hour of motivational interviewing could pay for healthcare for nine stateless kids on the Burmese border for an entire year, and chances are excellent that the patient's still going to keep eating/smoking/drinking/drugging, so screw it. Screw it.

The hematemetic woman died. If the doctor had been nicer, more compassionate, she still would have died. The floppy yellow baby died too, and the labor nurse didn't bat an eye. "How do you feel, after driving through the jungle for three hours to deliver a dead baby?" I asked her afterwards. "How do you feel knowing that this could have been prevented with a little bit more education, a little bit more public health?" She considered. "This is how these people live," she said. "They are poor, they have no education." "But how do you feel?" I asked, desperate. She thought for a moment. "I have to pee." Does it matter, that this suffering no longer matters to her?

I want to believe that compassion as I understand it is important. I want to believe that words and touch can heal injured bodies and souls, and that this type of healing matters somehow. But maybe I hold this belief because I crave compassion and loving kindness in my own life, because my human imperfection manifests itself in this particular way with this particular want. Have I been indulgent all this time?

I crash-landed back in Hanover in mid-August, several days late to school and several circles deep in Disparity Hell. I shoved my Schwartz notebooks under a pile of textbooks and left them there. I slept fitfully, dreaming in a fiery jumble of Thai and

English about broken bodies. I resolved to stop wasting my time on cushy intellectualism, to focus my energy on learning about disease processes so that I could become the sort of physician who could swoop in and rectify some of the intolerable physical sufferings in Umphang. Icky-squishy feelings be damned; I was going to memorize every last word of Harrison's. But after several weeks of immersion in the familiarly numbing routine of medical school, the immediacy of Disparity Hell faded. I ascended without hardly realizing it, progressed to purgatory, and emerged, dulled.

This undertaking has generated more questions than answers. I'm not sure how to define compassion, how to teach it, how to create a healthcare system that values it. I still fear that my empathetic capacity will be overwhelmed by the depth and breadth of my patients' suffering. I can't figure out how to sleep soundly while I work to reconcile the disparity between the two healthcare systems that I know.

But while I can't make any formal recommendations about how to teach compassion, I have come away with some ideas about how I intend to learn it. I believe that I'll learn best by example, so I'm seeking out role models who are known for their empathy and capacity for deep thinking. I think I'll have the most hope of holding on to my deepest self if I have a community of co-workers and co-learners to keep me accountable, even in trying circumstances. To build a culture of accountability, we have to be able to dialogue about compassion and caring. So I'm talking about this with everyone who will listen, and asking difficult questions when I see other students and doctors fall short. I hope that they will do the same for me.

It ends and starts again in a large rural hospital on the Vermont–New Hampshire border. I'm crouched at a patient's bedside watching closely as a palliative care doctor speaks with this dying man. She sits, pulls her chair close, puts her hand on his. I store away the words she chooses to bypass his defenses, study his face when something she says hits home. I note the pull in my chest. My definition of compassion isn't complete, not yet. But I have an idea of what it looks like, what it sounds like, what it feels like. This is the work I plan to do for the rest of my life.

MEGAN L. | United States

Notes to the Powers That Be

Hi Dr. W,

I showed up to clinic this morning in time to review my first patient's medical history. I was surprised to see "Homosexual Behavior" on the problem list, nestled between "Gout" and "Hyperlipidemia." My first thought was that this might have been entered as a risk factor for sexually transmitted infections (STIs). I have to say I'm not crazy about the practice of using sexual identity as a risk factor, but as someone who has worked as a sexual health counselor for five years, I understand the research behind it and that the current system might have merit.

So, eager to find an explanation, I dug deeper through the chart. "Homosexual behavior" had been present on the patient's problem list for over a year. There was no reference to any STI or relevant medical condition. I tried to think of other reasons that might explain the documentation but nothing came up. Even if there were some reason, risk factors like these belong in the social history, not on the problem list.

I wrote a strongly worded progress note and included in my plan, removing the diagnosis from the problem list. The manner in which it was documented is troubling, and even more so, that there was even an option to document it in this way (there was an associated international classification of diseases (ICD) code). The matter has since been rectified and I am glad, for the patient's sake, that the diagnosis was removed, but as a health-care system, we must continue to strive to do better.

Best,

Dr. Mikey

DR. MIKEY | United States

Lessons from the ED

- There is no time limit when a patient needs you to listen.
- Let your patients feel heard. The success of medications might hinge on it.
- Yes, patients presenting to the emergency department for non-urgent reasons may be frustrating but sometimes, the ED can be a vehicle to reach out to, and counsel patients that were previously not accessing primary care.
- Don't let bias motivate your actions; check your assumptions and be diligent in your investigations.

ANNA D. | Canada

Time

As a runner, time has long been both my greatest friend and adversary, and the clock in which it is embodied has served as an honest telltale of strength and effort. However, in this past year, I have come to know time in a new, intimate manner. Rotating through all medical specialties at a single hospital, I've been part of the time of birth, hand delivering a baby, as well as the time of death, after giving chest compressions in the Emergency Room. I've counseled patients on timing of insulin for diabetes and

medication for other chronic conditions, and discussed prognosis time in the face of a new cancer diagnosis. I've become well
versed in "time outs" before beginning an operation, and grown
privy to the time of the 9 p.m. meal (free dinner from the cafeteria's leftovers), time of an eighty-hour workweek, time with
patients, family, and friends.

Time is the ultimate currency, one we don't know how much
of we have, only that it is a precious treasure. I am excited to finish this year with renewed humility for the essence of time, as I
continue to pursue a career in neurosurgery and a mission to accompany patients in their fight against, or journey with, the clock.

FAITH R. | United States

The Doctor's Doctor

"You're too personable to go into radiology." It was clear the nurse
practitioner had been debating whether or not to tell me this and
had finally decided to spit it out. It wasn't the first time I had
heard this sentiment, and I couldn't help but smile. Thanking her
for her concern, I told her I believed I would be a nicer person in
the long run by doing radiology. She chuckled.

I came into medical school with an ambivalent attitude. All
through college, I took pre-med courses out of interest, but also
studied French and chemistry, hoping to find something to do
with my life other than medicine. However, by the end of senior
year, I had not devised any other concrete game plan, and so I
took the path of least resistance and went to medical school. I
was wholly convinced that I could make it through these four
years of undergraduate medical training, it was merely a question of whether I wanted to or not.

Upon entering medical school, I thought that I wanted to be
a family physician, a jack of all trades taking care of patients and
their families from cradle to grave. My romanticized vision of an

ideal physician was an antiquated one, of a beloved nineteenth-century village doctor riding on horseback with her medical bag in tow to check in on patients she had known all her life. Though in the twenty-first century I would not be on horseback, I still envisioned embedding myself in a community and knowing patients so well that we would be a large part of each other's lives.

I threw myself into primary care and family medicine interest group activities during my pre-clinical years. On paper, family medicine remained my ideal specialty choice. Yet, when shadowing a family physician, I developed a sneaking suspicion that I did not enjoy being in clinic, where I constantly felt rushed, stressed, and unfulfilled. I was also told that while I could remain quiet and shy in my personal life, I needed to develop a second persona for the hospital that was louder and more outgoing if I wanted to do well. Hearing this advice made me uncomfortable, but I forged on and, though it drained me, did my best to make myself more talkative. Although I felt uneasy and unsatisfied with these early clinical experiences, I chalked these feelings up to my particular shadowing clinic being too busy, and trekked on with my pre-clinical studies, convincing myself to wait until third-year clerkships to fully experience family medicine.

I had my family medicine rotation early on in third year, right after my radiology elective. Unfortunately, I reaffirmed my suspicion that I disliked being in clinic. I disliked not knowing whom I was going to see in the next exam room and did not jive well with my supervising residents and attendings. Furthermore, I disliked repeatedly counseling patients about hypertension, smoking, and diabetes, conversations I had thought would be the highlight of my day. I was disheartened, disappointed, and discouraged. How could there be such a huge disconnect between what I believed I would like doing and what I actually liked doing?

Also, while I had started medical school thinking that getting through would be a matter of whether I wanted to do it or not, I found that this was not the case. I had been struggling academically and felt like the rug had been pulled out from under me when I barely squeaked by on the United States Medical Licensing Examination (USMLE) Step one exam. It was no longer a matter of merely applying myself, because here I was, trying my best and wanting to learn and succeed, and yet still falling short. My cavalier attitude coming into medical school had long since been checked. And now the sliver of hope that I had hung onto during the first two years, believing that somehow I might end up liking family medicine after all, had vanished. That ever-lingering question of, "Is this worth it?" now had a blunt answer: "No."

I met with one of my deans, who encouraged me to "hang in there," believing that I had not seen enough of clinicals to make an informed decision about whether or not to leave medical school. I am grateful that I heeded her advice and was able to experience enjoying rotations that I thought I would dread, like surgery and OB/GYN, and disliking others, like pediatrics, I thought I would feel drawn to. Even though radiology was my first rotation, it was not until my last clerkship, in internal medicine, that I made the decision to pursue it. In a moment of clarity during a radiology lecture for medicine clerkship students, it dawned on me that I loved looking at imaging, and moreover, that I could be doing that all day. In addition, the radiology department made me feel like family—I had been working evenings in the radiology reading room for spending money, and had thoroughly enjoyed my interactions with the staff, residents, and attendings in the department. Not only did I like the work they did day-to-day, these people embraced me for who I was, shy and quiet as I could sometimes be, without asking me to change my personality. Ironically, I was even being told by others that I was "too personable" for radiology.

I felt a renewed sense of purpose that I had previously lacked in medical school. This new drive allowed me to look forward to my future and to strive for a new goal, to become a radiologist. One often hears, jokingly, that a radiologist is the "doctor's doctor," in the sense of being a consultant who makes a lot of patients' diagnoses through imaging. I intend to extend this moniker in a different direction; I intend not only to be a consultant to other doctors, but also to look out for other doctors' well-being. I have seen many ugly interactions in the hospital during my brief years of training, with people taking their anger and frustrations out on colleagues, residents, students, nurses, staff, or even patients, inciting a cascading effect that ultimately leads to poorer patient care. Yet I have also seen individuals who withstand the pressures of the hospital environment and instead lift up those working alongside them.

Towards the very end of my medical school training, I worked with an inspiringly kind neurosurgeon who believed that if he could absorb all the stress into himself instead of lashing out at others, then he could keep those around him in the OR or clinic in a better mood, and thus effect better patient care. I believe this neurosurgeon stood out for me by being such a caring individual in a field that, like radiology, is not necessarily known for having the friendliest physicians. I hope to emulate his qualities in my career as a radiologist, and as a "doctor's doctor" to spread happiness and kindness to those around me. Though I may or may not see patients on a regular basis, I still envision myself as a modern version of a nineteenth-century village doctor, with my horse and handbag traded in for scanners and picture archiving and communication systems (PACS), and my village comprising of other providers and caretakers working with me in the hospital.

MY-LINH N. | United States

Race-Based Medicine

"No one ever listens. Y'all just poke and prod. I have been telling them for years that these don't work for me!"

"That hurt! Get that away from me!" By the third day, I knew better than to urge Ms. Williams to let us take her blood pressure. It seemed like the nurse had also come to that same understanding. He quickly took off the blood pressure cuff and walked away — Ms. W. would not get any push back from him.

"How was your night?"

"I couldn't sleep all night."

"What has been keeping you up?"

"You know I don't sleep at night. I am afraid I am going to stop breathing."

"Did you feel short of breath?"

"I am always short of breath!"

She had had it with me. She tore off half of the muffin that was in front of her and pulled her breakfast tray closer. That was my cue to leave.

"I will be back later to the finish the exam"

It was much brighter outside her room, I had to give myself a few seconds to adjust. Ms. W. always kept her shades down. It was 8:30 a.m. — I had to hustle to get back for morning rounds.

"People say we don't have welfare! She is welfare! There is no way I am giving that woman a pacemaker. She is not going to come for follow-up, and she is not going to take her medications. She is not even that bright. That's the issue with all of them." Dr. M. was the cardiologist we had consulted to evaluate whether a defibrillator or a pacemaker could or should be placed in Mrs. W. He didn't like her or this idea very much. But all I could think about was how black people and women were less likely than whites and men respectively, to undergo a cardiac catheterization or a coronary artery bypass graft when admitted to the hospital for chest pain or a heart attack. It was statistically proven that interventions that could have been life-saving were not done because of inherent racial and gender bias.

"Also start her on Hydralazine-Isosorbide dinitrate (H-I). Those drugs work better in African Americans. We practice evidence-based medicine here." Dr. M. chuckled to himself as he got up to leave. He had walked in during the middle of morning rounds so we had to take a few seconds to figure out where we had left off.

Later that afternoon, I went to check on Ms. W. We still hadn't gotten a blood pressure on her but the nurse was able to convince her to wear the nasal cannula. Ms. W. was in florid heart failure when we admitted her. She had stopped going to her adult day care and was not taking her medications. She was sleeping on her belly, her forehead pressed against the wall— flexing her head just enough to keep her airways open. Her daughters had arrived by then; one worked as a nurse and the other was a home health aide. Both took care of their mother. Despite having her children in the medical field, Ms. W. did not trust white coats.

"Please don't take offense when Mummy is short with you."

"She just never trusted doctors after Nana's sister passed away because the emergency room wouldn't admit colored people."

Ms. W. was born into an America where medical treatment was available to black people only in certain locations, and only after all the white people were treated. American laws prohibited white female nurses from taking care of black men. She had lived through a time when the advent of segregated hospitals was a massive step forward in equalizing care.

"And Uncle Felix died at the house from diphtheria. Cold and blue, choked out of the air. They couldn't find a doctor that would help him. Mummy never got to see him."

US doctors and scientists created a racial inferiority mythology. Some alleged that blacks constituted the missing link between apes and man. And others suggested discontinuing relief to the poor because it perpetuated inferior racial stock and undermined social progress.

"Mummy doesn't go to the doctors for anything. She didn't even come to the City Hospital when she gave birth." I informed the daughters about Cardiology's decision. They didn't have a rebuttal, there were no pleas to reconsider. They were more concerned about the hematoma, the pool of blood, which had collected under their mom's forehead, the site where Ms. W. had pulled out her IVs a couple of days ago. I apologized for the appearance of the arm. We didn't cover much else.

The African American Heart Failure Trial (AHEFT)—H-I trial for my purposes here—was a "multicenter, double-blinded, parallel group, randomized, placebo-controlled trial," meaning that the highest level of integrity and a true application of the scientific method were adhered to when conducting this study. This trial categorically showed that using the H-I combination saved African American lives: for every thirteen people treated, this drug saved one life, an astounding finding in modern medicine where for many other drugs, one needed to treat hundreds of patients to see any benefit.

Trials like these are a huge achievement for Western medicine. There was a point in the dark days of Western medicine when physicians created a lexicon of "Negro diseases" and alternate physiological mechanisms based on race—chronic leprosy (theory that black skin, facial features, body odor, relative insensitivity to pain in black people was due to a congenital form of leprosy), Hypochondriasis, Drapetomania (disease of the mind that induces a slave to run away from service), Cachexia Africana. Scientific legitimization to these findings allowed African Americans to continue to suffer excess morbidity and mortality. And today, with the purest application of the scientific method, we have arrived at an enlightened age where science is a force for healing of all people.

We spent evening rounds figuring out a way to safely discharge Ms. W. There was not a lot that we could do for her in the hospital and she definitely didn't want to stay. We arranged for all her medications to be sorted and colored-coded into packs for her morning and night doses. She would no longer have to think about when to take which medication. We set up appointments for her with her primary care provider, the cardiologist, and the nutritionists. Social work was also going to check in with her after discharge to help set up transportation to the office visits and a health care worker would be coming to help Ms. W. around the house. My attending was insistent on having support systems in place that would help patients succeed after they left the hospital and decrease their chance of readmission. "This is where healthcare needs to focusing. We need to discuss the inherent inequality in our system," she said as we finished up our work for the day.

Sadly, Ms. W. was back in the hospital in two weeks and we were rehashing the pacemaker conversation again. It turns out that the h-1 trail correlated race with genetic variation and did not take into account that the benefits seen might have been due to treating the underlying causes of heart failure, not an intrinsic physiologic process in a specific racial group. The study also compared two sets of African Americans and concluded that the drug was beneficial in African Americans. h-1 does work, but I am not sure how well it works.

Anyway, Ms. W. was back because she was not taking her medications again. We restarted Ms. W. on the h-1 combination. But this time her heart, unable to pump appropriately, had flooded her lungs, choking her, and turning her cool and blue. She needed to go to the icu and be put on a ventilator.

In medicine, race is often used to account for the differences in biological outcomes and the risk of diseases. Race labels serve as diagnostic indicators and have a bearing on the prescription of specific drugs. Researchers use race as a marker for biology. But can non-scientific ideas like race, which is socially defined by the physical criterion, be used as a scientific category? Genomic studies have proven the insignificance of the old parameters of classification like skin color, hair texture, or skull size. There is no scientific legitimization of the concept of race. So we intentionally blur the lines and turn sociological differences into physiologic ones when we practice race-based medicine. And we continue to take part in scientific racism, though the othering is much more subversive.

Ms. W. had an uneventful ICU stay and was discharged home, again with all the wrap around services in place. The nurses and doctors knew that she would be readmitted soon. And the next intern would have to start her on H-1 and quote to their attending the benefits of this treatment over other regimens.

SYED S. | United States

Stay Alert, Stay Alive

It wasn't until the second to last day of my four weeks shadowing a physician at a correctional facility that I saw those words painted over one of the many gates you needed to go through to get into the prison. It was hazard yellow on a chalky blue background, and my first reaction was disappointment. It paints prison as incredibly dangerous — and don't get me wrong, I'm sure it can be — but the people I've seen here strike me much more as people who made a poor choice along the way, be it gang violence, drugs, or sexual abuse. These infractions have strong cases for environmental causation, societal conditioning, poor mental health, and weak support structures.

While I realized there were indeed sociopaths in the world, the fear of these inmates seemed largely unfounded to me, after spending time with some of them. The elderly patient who happily let me stick a tube up his penis to drain his bladder, and still smiled warmly and wished me good luck in my studies wasn't someone I felt my life threatened by. The man who had been a drug dealer, and told me he would go right back to selling drugs when he got out because that was the only way he knew to support his wife and children, wasn't someone I feared. Rather, I respected his loyalty to his family, even if it cost him his own freedom. Similarly, although the man who was addicted to pain medication and had a broken jaw with residual nerve damage was a huge man, in talking to him, you could tell he just wanted to talk to someone who would try to understand him. Granted, he might also have wanted drugs, but he was equally a victim of drug addiction, which research has shown us is driven by the lack of productive socialization society perpetuates by ostracizing addicts.

My preceptor and I had a lot of conversations about the morality, ethics, and finances of not only prison as an institution, but also the medical care inmates should or should not have access to. We discussed the Zimbardo experiment, in which a university professor assigned each student the role of guard or prisoner. The students acting as guards embraced their power a little too much, jeering at and shaming the prisoners, who hadn't done anything wrong, but suffered mental breakdowns from the isolation and the abuse. The experiment stood today as a caution to the negative effects of excessive use of power on the human psyche. However, it seemed to me that the manner in which we ran prisons ignored this research, and without providing inmates with the skills and support systems to flourish in society, did more harm than good. It struck me that we all have the capacity to kill others, myself even more so as a doctor. We all have the capacity to be pushed to desperation that might drive us across legal lines. Some people actually do cross these lines, and are either never caught, or receive mild wrist slaps. Yet we brand the population that wasn't so lucky as "other," and subject them to a system that does not help them.

Stay alert. Stay alive. Stay humane. Find humility. Find empathy. Practice compassion. As we think about how we rehabilitate those who have broken the law, I hope we will let these words, and research, guide us.

IANNA H-M. | United States

Invisible Women

The consultation room is small, with just enough space to accommodate the gynaecology consultant, myself, and the individual patients that are to follow. The room has an examination
bed, a desk, and sink on the opposite corner. The windows are
covered, hiding the rays of the scorching African sun that burns
mid-summer. Gynaecology is my first clinical rotation for the
year. Having been placed at Mahatma Gandhi Memorial Hospital in Durban, South Africa, I looked forward to the knowledge and practical experience I would gain as I developed in the
medical profession.

Creeping through the door, two children appear, then behind
them a woman, clad in black material and a black scarf, deco-
rated with a kaleidoscope of patterns. In her arms is an infant,
not more than a year old.

When the consult begins, she awkwardly asks for an abortion. When we begin trying to estimate the gestational age by
date we approximate it to five weeks. In South Africa, since the
implementation of the Choice of Termination of Pregnancy Act
in 1997, abortion should be freely available to all women through
the first trimester, and thereafter only available under specific
circumstances, with stringency increasing as the gestational age
increases.

She is informed that she will have to return in a weeks' time as
the foetus is yet to be visible on the ultrasound, and is further
explained to that continuing with the abortion could pose a risk
to her life as an extra uterine pregnancy is yet to be excluded.

The tone in her voice changes. She pleads desperately: "I don't
think I will be able to come here again!" She goes on to explain
that if she prolongs this any longer her husband may become
aware of the pregnancy and then she will be forced to continue

with it. When she realises that her pleas are not being heard, she quickly hurries away. I silently pray she is able to attend her next appointment.

DAY FOUR | 11:08 A.M.
Her braids rest comfortably over her school attire. I assume no one knows she skipped school to come to the gynaecology out-patient department. She too asks for an abortion, however, un-like the previous patient, the petiteness of this sixteen-year-old only accentuates her abdominal distension when she removes her loosely fitting jersey. The ultrasound findings do not correlate with her history of having her last menstrual period three months ago; her gestational age is just over twenty weeks. Since abortion is no longer a possibility, she is counselled along her remaining options and is written a referral to the hospital psychologist.

She is silent, but the worry in her eyes screams of uncer-tainty and fear. Tears begin to roll down her cheeks, and she is reminded by my senior not to attempt to contact illegal abortion providers — but in her mind, it may be her only option.

DAY EIGHT| 10:05 A.M.
The ward round began exactly at 8:30 a.m. The ward is com-prised of three large cubicles, all adjacent to one another. Venti-lation is poor, and this, combined with high temperatures, makes it almost unbearable to be in. The diagnoses are just as varied as the room's racial and socioeconomic demographics, which closely mimics South Africa's.

When we approach the bed of the final patient to be seen, I begin wondering what exactly could be wrong with her. She looks young, no older than her late teens. Her hair is long, and she is covered by a thin purple blanket. The consultant's review of the patient does not provide much further information, and as the round concludes, a colleague and I stall to quickly read her file. The file reveals that she had ingested rodent poison in an attempt to induce an abortion. From her initial examination and blood results, she was lucky to be alive.

Growing up in a religious and conservative background, sensitive topics dealing with sex were seldom discussed. I chose to pursue a career in medicine during my high school years—I yearned to be part of the medical forensics teams I idolized from television. These dreams carried me through many difficult years of schooling and studying. (As many can testify, for a South African of Indian origin, gaining a place at any medical university in South Africa is no easy task).

When I eventually entered the health care system as a medical student, I realised the public health care sector in South Africa was incomparable to the technologically savvy Western facilities I admired. I was shocked to see the reality of the statistics I was taught in school. My home province of KwaZulu-Natal had one the highest incidence rates of HIV in the world, and I witnessed women, specifically black South African women, suffer in a system that seemed to have been created to fail them.

When I began my third year of medical school, I was fortunate to attend a medical student conference that brought together more than a thousand students from over a hundred countries to discuss pertinent topics and themes related to medical student experiences and global health care. Naturally, I attended the sessions on sexual and reproductive health including HIV/AIDS, and during the segment on maternal health and access to safe abortion, I was enlightened on the global struggles women face in different regions of the world when it came to safe and legal abortion access. I reflected on my experiences and knowledge of South African abortion laws and I pondered why, in a country that has been praised to have one of the most progressive legislations on abortion in the world, women are still dying from unsafe abortion procedures.

When I began to research abortion-related topics in South Africa, I learnt that political agendas, personal opinions, cultural views, and stigma were interwoven to oppress women. I also wrestled internally with my religious views and what my professional ethos ought to be. I realised that as a future medical professional, I had to behave in a manner that is exactly that, professional, and in a manner that was non-judgmental. I needed to be able to provide holistic health care and meet all my patients' needs; if I could not do that, then maybe medicine wasn't for me after all.

When people advocate for abortion rights, they advocate for more than just that: they advocate for women's total autonomy over their own bodies and for a world in which women are empowered to make independent decisions about their lives, about where they can drive, what they can earn. Nelson Mandela said, "a nation cannot be free until its women are free." Women should be free to access quality healthcare, but in many parts of the world, the opposite is true, as women are ostracised and incarcerated for attempting to access safe abortion services, and in many cases pushed to their deaths as a result.

When I look into my future in the medical profession, I see myself committed to improving our global health care systems. Every maternal life matters and women should have the freedom to exercise their rights regarding their own bodies in an environment free from bias and judgement.

VIKAR S. | South Africa

Three Days in the ICU

While preparing my application to medical school, I shadowed palliative care consultants, volunteered at a hospice, wrote my undergraduate dissertation on the influence of spirituality and religious beliefs on the anticipatory grief of the terminal patient, and read hundreds of books and articles on end-of-life topics. Back then, I was convinced that the best example of true holistic care was palliative care (which made it my dream specialty). Intensive care, on the other hand, was the antithesis of holistic medicine and was hence, an area I would never dare to consider. But one spring day, during my first year of medical school, something extraordinary happened during an ordinary lecture on hypoxia. The lecturer, a consultant in intensive care medicine, while commenting on something apparently unrelated, suggested that "there cannot be a good provision of intensive care without the integration of palliative care," and that "when the patient is facing death, palliative care must be a central part of his care plan." I remember those words vividly, as they captured my attention straight away: *Palliative care in intensive care? Was that even possible?* I needed to explore that further, and so I decided to contact the intensivist, who let me visit his unit for three days during the summer break.

In the weeks preceding my visit to the unit, to gain a more accurate understanding of the specialty, I read a lot about intensive care medicine: numerous articles as well as books, including *The Textbook of Post-ICU Medicine, Delirium in Critical Care* by Valerie Page and Wesley Ely, or *Through the Valley of Shadows* by Samuel Brown, as well as numerous articles. My preconceived ideas (built upon many other readings over the years) had been very focused on the mistaken perception that what usually happens in the ICU is the opposite of what good end-of-life care should be. Consequently, I was wary and skeptical about what I was going to encounter in the unit. Would I see patients dying, connected to machines and tubes, surrounded by noises and without their family members nearby? Would I enter into an ICU full of alarms, without windows, and where time passed without references? How would someone like me feel in there, someone who saw palliative care as having nothing to do with ICUs?

To my surprise, my first impression of the ICU was very positive: the ward was beautiful and spacious, and the rooms had enormous windows facing a garden. I had two contrasting feelings: on the one hand, I had entered into a place where alertness was palpable — patients were critically ill and closely monitored — but on the other hand, I also felt a certain peace in the unit. The space I was in was full of natural light, with clocks in each room that enabled patients and family members track the passage of time, and no monitors or annoying alarms beeping constantly.

After an initial briefing with the intensivist, I attended a meeting with other physicians. It was there I learnt that two of the patients in the unit were dying, and that the palliative care team was with the families in the rooms. I also discovered that the chaplain was coming later in the morning to provide spiritual support. Somewhat surprised, the idea that perhaps palliative and intensive care were not so antithetic after all again crossed my mind. I had three days to see if it was indeed true.

During the first ward round with the consultant and three junior doctors, I noticed that patients were accompanied by their families or friends without restrictions, and was pleased to see that nurses and physicians alike openly conveyed understanding of the difficulty of patients' situations, offering support and compassionate care. I also noticed that the physicians talked to the patients — conscious or not — with respect at all times, letting them know who they were and what was going to happen, asking them permission to carry out the physical examination, and covering them immediately to preserve their privacy. I enjoyed witnessing this, because these aspects of care are essential elements in the humanization of the medical practice, and are as important as, if not more important than, the technical knowledge. While witnessing the physicians' interaction with the patients, I noticed that their work combined intellectual, practical, and reflective skills. They spent a considerable amount of time in each room, observing and examining the patient. They asked questions when possible, thought systematically, and shared their ideas with other colleagues.

Even more than the intellectual challenge of the ICU, it was the respect that physicians conveyed to the patient at all times, the constant efforts to preserve the patient's dignity, and the inclusion of the patient and/or the patient's family when decisions had to be taken that appealed to me. Even in the most technological of hospital wards, treating the patient as a human being rather than as a pathology was possible. Indeed, palliative and intensive care were not so antithetic after all.

On my last day, one of the consultants invited me to be present in a family meeting for a dying patient. Given my interest in palliative care, I had read extensively on end-of-life topics. But being there with the intensivist and the family allowed me more tangibly appreciate the complexity of those conversations, and the importance of delivering bad news with empathy. I listened as the intensivist, with both her words and silences, conveyed compassion and presence to the family.

Those three days in the ICU marked a turning point in my medical and personal journey: they broadened my horizons, opened my mind, and made me reflect extensively on the care of the critically ill patients and what practicing holistic medicine truly involves. Both palliative care and intensive care aim to relieve patients' unnecessary suffering, and accompany them in the process of finding meaning and purpose in life, and in dying.

BARBARA S. | United Kingdom

CONCLUSION

As I have worked on this anthology, I have gained an even deeper appreciation for the process of becoming—the folding and unfolding, doing and undoing. Over the past months, reflections have poured in at times, and trickled at others. I have gone through stages of doubt, confidence, uncertainty, and resoluteness, wondering how—or if—the anthology would emerge. If I'm honest, there were periods I only kept going because I had involved too many people—contributors, loved ones, strangers turned angels—and I didn't want to disappoint them or make their efforts for naught. Through compiling this anthology, I have learned that sometimes, perfect is the enemy of good—perfect is the enemy of process.

Medical training is not perfect. It never has been and, although I hate to admit it, it probably never will be. As I have joined my own reflections with my colleagues' and drawn parallels between our journeys to Doctor and the journey to a finished book, I have come to accept that at no point will there be a finish line. Life—and all its compartments—is a work in progress, a perpetual process. The book you have in your hands is not a finished product, just as medical training, and the philosophy around it, are not final iterations. Many stories and voices are missing from the pages of *Human*, just as many considerations are missing from the current medical training system.

The conversation around medical trainee wellness has intensified all over the world since I started working on this collection. I have heard the themes contained in *Human*, echoed across both academic and nonacademic platforms. These conversations have been messy—and rightly so, life is incapable of sterility—but we must not bury them or chalk them up to "millennial whining." Feet genuinely hurt in ill-fitting shoes. I hope the reflections in *Human* add meaningfully to the evolving conversation of how we train our doctors. We cannot say as a society, "This has always worked," when reality is telling us otherwise, when things that have been hidden are now coming to light.

The current conversation about medical training needs to involve all members of society, not just institutions that have traditionally overseen medical training, like hospitals and medical schools. As we debate about rising healthcare costs, universal coverage, and healthcare access, let us not forget the people that sustain the system, the people on whose backs the system is borne. A sustainable system must steward all its resources responsibly—physical, economic, and human. We must not leave one out of the picture. Again, as life often is, the future will likely be messy, but move, we must. Perfect is the enemy of process.

On a clinical rotation last year, I met lovely nurse, June Garen, whose son, like me, was in his third year of medical school. She was incredibly kind to me and made me feel seen, a welcome luxury for a third-year medical student. In one of our discussions, I mentioned this book to her and was pleasantly surprised to see an email from her sometime after. She had written a letter to her son, to help him find his way as he figured out his own training process. Although I intended *Human* to contain reflections from current medical trainees, I was drawn to June's letter, because it highlighted the fact that medical trainees exist in a larger social setting, that medical trainees come from a place, and are supported through, and to, places by loved ones. These loved ones are dragged along with us for better or worse, and so ought to get a seat at the table. I therefore leave you with June's words and the reminder to not let perfect hinder process as we journey.

Dear Jonathan,

As you launch off into clinical rotations, I have had some thoughts to share while I mull over your journey. These mental meanderings come from both a mother's and a nurse's perspective.

I know that medical school is an endeavor that is definitely not undertaken casually. Your determination and commitment to not only the application process, but also each year of your studies, has humbled me. You have survived and excelled through the traps and snares of the first two years. Now, your reward consists of being ejected into the world of hospitals and clinics to care for real patients.

Recently, sitting together enjoying some lovely eats on a rainy New Orleans afternoon, you looked at me and said, "It got real today." You told me the story of your patient, who you had grown to really like and enjoy. She had recently found out that she was terminally ill. My heart broke a little for you because, after all, you will always be my son and I hate to see you sad. We spoke that soggy afternoon of feelings of sadness, frustration, and inadequacy. We also talked about how different the real-life journey is from that in the safe arena of a standardized patient. We spoke of the gift that is given to us in our professions; that of helping people manage the end of life adventure with dignity, respect, and kindness. Finally, we both acknowledged the gift given to us by constantly facing illness, injury, and death: the awareness that life and good health may be very temporary and thus embracing both with a grateful heart is imperative.

So here are a few pearls of wisdom for you to hold tightly as you meander along in your vocation:

Always start your day with a clear mind and sound focus. I liken it to being a bullfighter entering into the ring; you need to stay alert and pay attention at all times.

Be kind. Let me repeat this, be kind. You never know what people hear or remember, but they will remember how you made them feel. They will respond best to respect and kindness. You will most likely always be your harshest critic . . . so, be kind to yourself, too.

Not every patient can be saved, but you can always be a healer.

Plan to be political; it is part of advocating for your patients. You live on the frontlines; policy makers and politicians do not.

Mistakes can be vicious, but effective, teachers.

Allow people to help you. Don't be afraid to ask questions. Many folks are intimidated by the letters you will soon sign at the end of your name. Don't fall prey to the notion that MD stands for "modern deity."

Patients may be challenging, but without them, our professions would cease to exist. They are the center of our universe. Remember that all of your patients are important and deserving of respect. Set that tone for the rest of your team, too.

Don't be afraid to set limits and boundaries. You deserve the chance to rest and recuperate.

As hard as this may be to accept, the patient has goals which may supersede the ones that you would like to set.

Finally, never forget that it is an honor and privilege to care for people at their most vulnerable moments.

Always remember that I am endlessly proud of you.

Love,
Mom

ACKNOWLEDGMENTS

A tribute to my village

Compiling *Human* has been a lesson in patience and thanksgiving. Patience, because projects often don't pan out as linearly as one might have hoped, and thanksgiving, because throughout the journey to getting this collection to your hands, people have proven themselves to be golden.

I would like to thank my colleagues and contributors, who sent in reflections from their respective countries with votes of confidence that a project like *Human* was an important undertaking. Special thanks to Kathleen Reich for collecting quotes (the anonymized ones that began most chapters) from her classmates and making them available to me. This book would literally be empty (or at best, ten pages long) without you all. Thank you for your patience with me, as timelines were extended and updates sparse.

To the strangers turned angels, you have put me in an almost constant state of awe at human kindness. Dr. Joe O'Donnell, thank you for reading my thirty-seven-page book proposal and going out of your way to see this book come to fruition. Dan Berger, I have told several people of the incredibly kind immigration lawyer in Northampton, Massachusetts, who spent hours helping me navigate complex US immigration laws. Your warmth and generosity were highlights of this process. Megan Reid, thank you for showing a clueless newbie how to write a book proposal. Thank you too, for reading the thirty-seven-page book proposal of a friend of a friend. Pamela Wible, your energy and devotion to preventing medical trainee suicides are incredible. Thank you for giving me the boost I needed, and for bringing me into the "17 in 2017" group. Thank you to all members of the 17 in 2017 group, for your insights and support. Dr. Danielle Ofri, you responded to an email from a random medical student. Thank you for your insights and for your work to increase the influence of the humanities in medicine. Sam Shem, you are golden for your patience as I repeatedly shifted deadlines under the weight of my other responsibilities. Thank you for consistently lending your voice to increasing humanism in medical training. To everyone who shared a post about the anthology on social media and encouraged friends to submit reflections, thank you.

To my personal hype people, thank you for love and support and continual hype—your girl needed it. Mom and Dad, thank you for letting me find my own way in life, even when it differed from yours. Thank you for the encouragement, the sacrifices and the love. Feyi, I'd choose you over again to be my big brother. I love you dearly. Thank you for always going ahead, for working hard and loving generously. To my cousins, thank you for the laughs and cheerleading. Lola, thank you for being a true sister. To the ladies of "No new friends," whom I have known since I was 10, you are friends if there ever were some. Thank you for inspiring me with your words and your own journeys. Jimi, your unwavering belief in me is quite incredible. Thank you. My Mount Holyoke sisters, you are the real deal. Thank you for always celebrating one person's triumphs as all of ours. Tomisin, my adopted big sister, thank you for encouraging the dream when it started; my adopted little sister, Rike, thank you for bringing joy, and for praying (#MiracleMay). To my Geisel family, thank you for always asking how the book was going and how I was doing. Vanessa, thank you for hooking me up with Megan and for your thoughts and time on the cover. You are golden. Dr. Pinto-Powell, throughout medical school, you encouraged me to keep writing. Thank you for being a dependable support. To my Tuck friends, thank you for taking my dreams in yours.

Richard Pult, my first editor, thank you for taking a chance on this anthology, and for offering this woman a dotted line to sign her name on. Thank you for your emails, advice, and edits. Without you, this book might just have been yet another file on my computer. Amanda Dupuis, thank you for picking up, so gracefully and with such kindness, where Richard left off.

If I have left anyone out, it is not for lack of gratitude. I have simply been blessed with more wonderful people than my brain can recollect in one sitting. Thank you all for being part of this journey. You kept me accountable and kept me moving. And of course, big thanks to the One who inspires dreams larger than one can imagine.